CW01433078

Isom(

Exercises

The Ultimate Guide to Isometric Exercises for Muscle Building

(A User Manual for Your Mind & the Ultimate Guide to Mental Toughness)

Jack Brown

Published By **Percy Clint**

Jack Brown

Isometric Exercises: The Ultimate Guide to Isometric Exercises for Muscle Building (A User Manual for Your Mind & the Ultimate Guide to Mental Toughness)

ISBN   978-0-9949563-9-2

Legal & Disclaimer

Table Of Contents

Chapter 1: Understanding Muscle Engagement In Isometrics

Muscle Contraction Types: Isometric, Isotonic, Isokinetic

Before delving into the specifics of isometric sporting occasions, its miles critical to recognise the idea of muscle contractions and the differing types that exist inside the realm of workout Understanding those muscle contraction sorts will provide valuable insights into how isometric physical video video games paintings and their particular benefits.

Muscle Contraction Types

1. Isometric Contraction:

Isometric contractions arise whilst muscle mass generate tension with none alternate in period, resulting in a static, steady function. During an isometric exercising, the muscle agencies settlement; however there may be no visible motion within the joints. An outstanding example of an isometric contraction is pushing in opposition to an immovable object, which incorporates in search of to push a wall. The muscle groups have interaction, but the wall does now not pass. This static nature of isometric sports activities lets in for focused muscle activation, making them ideal for power education and stability improvement.

2. Isotonic Contraction:

Isotonic contractions incorporate muscle adjustments in duration at the same time as generating anxiety. There are   types of isotonic contractions:

Concentric Contraction: In this sort of contraction, the muscle shortens because it contracts in opposition to resistance. For example, all through a bicep curl, the bicep muscle shortens as you boost the burden inside the route of your shoulder.

Eccentric Contraction: Eccentric contractions arise while the muscle lengthens because it contracts in competition to resistance. Using the identical bicep curl instance, the eccentric contraction takes location as you lower the weight backpedal slowly, resisting the pressure of gravity.

Isotonic contractions are fundamental to traditional weight training sports, contributing to muscle improvement, flexibility, and standard motion skillability.

three. Isokinetic Contraction:

Isokinetic contractions are characterized by using everyday muscle pace within the path of the movement. Specialized machine, along with isokinetic machines, is frequently used to manipulate the rate and resistance. These machines provide variable resistance to in form the character's attempt, making sure that the muscle contracts at a consistent speed irrespective of the completed stress.

Isokinetic physical sports activities are masses a great deal much less not unusual in conventional exercise settings, thru and massive utilized in physical treatment and rehabilitation settings because of the managed nature of the moves, decreasing the risk of damage.

Isometric Exercises and Muscle Contraction Types

Isometric wearing sports activities regularly recognition on isometric contractions, wherein the muscle generates anxiety without seen movement. By maintaining a tough and speedy characteristic or maintaining a particular posture, isometric bodily activities undertaking and decorate focused muscle companies efficaciously. The static nature of isometrics allows for a sustained, excessive muscle engagement, main to muscle recruitment and improvement.

It's vital to word that whilst isometric bodily sports excel in certain additives, incorporating masses of contraction sorts proper into a nicely-rounded health routine can lead to finish muscle development, superior joint balance, and extra appropriate commonplace fundamental performance. Understanding the versions among isometric, isotonic, and isokinetic contractions permits human beings to tailor their workout physical games to their precise health desires and needs, optimizing their exercise routine for advanced effects.

Targeting Specific Muscle Groups

One of the important factor benefits of isometric bodily video games is their ability to goal precise muscle corporations with precision. By keeping static positions and that specialize in muscle engagement, humans can isolate and enhance particular muscle tissues, developing a properly-balanced and centered exercising regular. Here's a breakdown of approaches isometric sports can effectively purpose numerous muscle organizations:

1. Upper Body Muscles:

Chest: Isometric wearing sports like wall push-usaor chest squeezes aim the pectoral muscular tissues, assisting to enhance pinnacle frame strength and decorate the appearance of the chest.

Shoulders: Isometric sports like shoulder presses or wall handstands cause the deltoid muscular tissues, essential to more potent and greater strong shoulders.

Back: Isometric bodily activities like plank versions and wall sits set off the again muscle tissues, together with the latissimus dorsi and trapezius, helping to enhance posture and decrease again energy.

Arms: Isometric physical video games like static bicep curls or tricep extensions target the biceps and triceps, promoting arm electricity and definition.

2. Lower Body Muscles:

Quadriceps: Isometric bodily games like wall sits or static lunges purpose the quadriceps, most important to stepped forward leg power and stability.

Hamstrings: Isometric carrying activities like hamstring curls or bridge holds engage the hamstrings, supporting to enhance the lower back of the thighs.

Glutes: Isometric physical video games like glute bridges or chair squats goal the gluteal muscle mass, contributing to higher hip balance and common decrease body power.

Calves: Isometric physical sports like calf increases against a wall or stair engage the calf muscle groups, assisting in calf strength and definition.

three. Core Muscles:

Abdominals: Isometric sports activities like plank variations or hollow frame holds are fantastic for focused on the stomach muscle organizations, foremost to progressed middle electricity and balance.

Obliques: Isometric physical video video games like aspect plank variations help have interaction the oblique muscle mass, selling higher waist definition and rotational balance.

Lower Back: Isometric physical video games like Superman holds cause the lower over again muscle tissues, contributing to a more potent and greater resilient decrease decrease back.

four. Total Body Engagement:

Full-Body Plank: The conventional plank exercise engages more than one muscle agencies simultaneously, such as the middle, fingers, shoulders, and legs, making it an green standard-frame isometric exercising.

Bear Crawl: While in a quadruped position, barely hovering above the ground, shifting the opportunity arm and leg in sync engages the center, shoulders, and hips, presenting a entire-frame exercise.

By incorporating severa isometric physical video games that focus on particular muscle businesses, human beings can format a whole workout everyday that meets their fitness dreams. It's crucial to keep right shape and perform each exercising with controlled movements to maximise muscle engagement and reduce the chance of damage.

Preparing Your Workout Space

Before embarking for your isometric exercise journey, it's far essential to set the degree for a steady and effective workout. Preparing your exercise place ensures that you have the crucial environment and system to perform isometric carrying occasions effects and with maximum benefits. Here's a step-by way of way of-step manual to getting began:

1. Clear and Open Space:

Choose a properly-lit and spacious area in your workouts. Clear any barriers or tripping dangers to create a secure surroundings for motion. If feasible, use a committed place wherein you may perform your physical sports without interruptions.

2. Exercise Mat or Cushioned Surface:

Consider the use of an workout mat or a cushioned floor to provide useful resource and luxury at some stage in floor-based isometric physical activities. A mat also can help save you slipping and protect your joints from extra stress.

three. Proper Clothing:

Wear comfortable and breathable workout garb that allows for an entire range of movement. Avoid free-turning into garments that would intrude collectively together along with your actions or get stuck throughout physical activities.

4. Footwear:

Choose footwear that gives stability and manual on your particular workout. For many isometric physical sports, barefoot or minimalist footwear may be appropriate to assist maintain stability and proper foot positioning.

5. Water and Towel:

Have a water bottle nearby to live hydrated in some unspecified time in the future of your exercising. Keep a towel reachable to wipe away sweat and preserve a comfortable exercise surroundings.

6. Timer or Stopwatch:

For timed isometric physical games, use a timer or a stopwatch to tune the duration of each hold correctly. This enables you preserve consistency and regularly growth the time as you development.

7. Variations and Modifications:

Familiarize yourself with one-of-a-type isometric physical games and their variations to aim numerous muscle organizations correctly. This allows you to customize your physical video games based completely virtually to your health stage and goals.

8. Warm-Up and Cool-Down:

Prior to beginning your isometric wearing activities, carry out a dynamic warmness-as lots as put together your muscular tissues and joints for the workout. After your workout, engage in static stretching as a part of your cool-down recurring to promote flexibility and reduce muscle tension.

9. Exercise Guidance:

If you're new to isometric carrying sports or unsure about proper form and techniques, take into account searching for guidance from health experts or first-rate on-line belongings. Understanding the best posture and muscle engagement is essential to keep away from harm and maximize the blessings of each exercise.

10. Consistency and Progression:

Like any fitness recurring, consistency is prime to seeing improvements. Set realistic dreams and step by step increase the intensity and duration of your isometric physical video video games as you assemble strength and self assurance.

Remember that isometric physical video video games may be tailor-made to in form numerous health degrees, from beginners to advanced practitioners. With right training and a steady workout environment, you can embark on a fulfilling isometric schooling adventure that contributes to advanced strength, balance, and ordinary bodily properly-being.

Essential Equipment and Tools

Isometric bodily video video games are renowned for his or her simplicity and effectiveness, and genuinely one in every of their attractive components is they require minimal device. While many isometric wearing activities can be completed using truly your body weight, there are some crucial pieces of equipment and equipment that can decorate your isometric exercise revel in and add variety to your ordinary. Here are a number of the crucial element gadgets to hold in thoughts:

1. Exercise Mat:

An exercise mat offers a cushty and non-slip floor for floor-based totally definitely isometric sports activities sports. It gives cushioning in your knees, elbows, and splendid frame components in contact with the ground, reducing the danger of pain and injury.

2. Stability Ball:

Also known as an exercising or Swiss ball, a stability ball provides versatility in your isometric bodily video games. It allows you to have interaction extra muscular tissues for your middle, lower back, and legs on the identical time as performing numerous stability wearing events.

three. Resistance Bands:

Resistance bands are exquisite equipment for isometric training. They are to be had in severa ranges of resistance, allowing you to personalize the intensity of your carrying events. You can use resistance bands to goal precise muscle businesses, supplying everyday tension at some stage in isometric holds.

four. Yoga Blocks:

Yoga blocks can help in improving isometric sports activities and enhancing flexibility. They provide beneficial resource for deeper stretches and assist you preserve proper alignment for the duration of superb poses.

5. Pull-Up Bar:

If you're looking for to comprise top body isometric carrying activities like static chin-usaor hangs, a pull-up bar can be a valuable addition to your property fitness center. It gives a robust anchor for numerous top body exercises.

6. Timer or Stopwatch:

For timed isometric wearing sports activities, a timer or stopwatch is essential. It allows you track the duration of every preserve and preserve consistency on your sporting events. This allows you to little by little increase the time as you improvement for your fitness adventure.

7. Hand Grippers:

Hand grippers or grip strengtheners are useful for focused on forearm muscles and improving grip energy. They can be beneficial for isometric physical sports that encompass squeezing and maintaining devices.

8. Yoga Strap or Resistance Loop Bands:

Yoga straps or resistance loop bands are valuable equipment for increasing flexibility and enhancing variety of motion. They may be used to assist in positive stretches and isometric sports activities.

9. Wall or Doorway:

Walls and doorways can function anchor factors for severa isometric sports activities. They permit you to push or pull in competition to a solid surface to interact special muscle corporations efficiently.

Chapter 2: Isometric Exercises For Upper Body

Chest and Pectoral Exercises

Strengthening the chest and pectoral muscle businesses is vital for regular better frame energy and stability. Isometric sporting occasions provide an exquisite way to aim and engage those muscle tissues correctly. Below are a few isometric carrying activities particularly designed to art work the chest and pectoral muscle corporations:

1. Wall Push-Up Hold:

Stand managing a wall, approximately arm's length away, and vicinity your arms at the wall at shoulder height and shoulder-width aside.

Lean your body in advance barely, appealing your chest muscular tissues.

Hold this position for a predetermined time (e.G., 20-30 seconds).

Focus on retaining tension on your chest in the course of the hold.

2. Static Chest Squeeze:

Sit or stand at the side of your decrease once more at once, and convey your hands together inside the front of your chest.

Press your hands collectively firmly, attractive your chest muscles.

Hold the squeeze for a predetermined time (e.G., 20-30 seconds).

Keep your elbows regular with your shoulders and hold regular respiratory.

three. Wall Chest Press Hold:

Stand going through far from a wall and area your palms on the wall at shoulder peak and shoulder-width aside.

Position your body at an attitude to the wall, along side your palms prolonged immediately within the front of you.

Press your fingers firmly in competition to the wall, engaging your chest muscle organizations.

Hold this position for a predetermined time (e.G., 20-30 seconds).

4. Isometric Push-Up Hold:

Assume a push-up function along side your palms located barely wider than shoulder-width apart and your frame in a right away line from head to heels.

Lower your body halfway down, maintaining your elbows at a ninety-degree attitude.

Hold this function together together with your chest just above the ground for a predetermined time (e.G., 20-30 seconds).

Focus on retaining tension for your chest and middle at a few stage in the maintain.

five. Isometric Fly Hold:

Lie in your lower decrease lower back along side your knees bent and ft flat on the floor.

Hold a resistance band or towel among each hands, fingers extended out to the edges.

Squeeze the band or towel as when you have been performing a fly motion, attractive your chest muscles.

Hold the squeeze for a predetermined time (e.G., 20-30 seconds).

6. Isometric Chest Press (with resistance band or wall):

Stand going via a wall or join a resistance band to a robust anchor factor.

Hold the band or wall with both fingers at chest height.

Press your hands in advance, appealing your chest muscle corporations.

Hold the clicking for a predetermined time (e.G., 20-30 seconds) at the same time as keeping tension to your chest.

Important Considerations:

Maintain right form ultimately of every isometric exercise to save you strain and harm.

Breathe little by little and avoid protective your breath within the course of the holds.

Start with shorter hold times and little by little increase the length as your strength improves.

Perform those wearing sports as part of a nicely-rounded better body exercise ordinary that still consists of wearing occasions for different muscle corporations.

Incorporating the ones isometric chest and pectoral sports into your health recurring can bring about multiplied top body energy, improved posture, and additional appropriate ordinary higher body stability. As with any workout software application, consistency and proper execution are key to engaging in the favored effects. If you're new to isometric sports activities or have any health issues, keep in mind consulting a health expert to make sure that your workout plan aligns together with your individual desires and goals.

Shoulder and Deltoid Exercises

Strengthening the shoulders and deltoid muscles is essential for better body power, balance, and traditional shoulder health. Isometric sporting activities offer an effective manner to cause and have interaction the shoulders, assisting to enhance their electricity and endurance. Below are some isometric physical sports mainly designed to work the shoulder and deltoid muscular tissues:

1. Isometric Shoulder Press:

Stand tall collectively together with your feet shoulder-width aside and hands bent at ninety degrees, forming a goalpost characteristic.

Push your fingers upwards in competition to an immovable object, together with a wall, door frame, or resistance band anchored above you.

Engage your shoulders and deltoids as you press in opposition to the resistance.

Hold this function for a predetermined time (e.G., 20-30 seconds) on the identical time as preserving tension to your shoulders.

2. Static Shoulder Abduction:

Stand collectively together with your arms at your sides and hands coping with your body.

Slowly improve your arms out to the edges, retaining them parallel to the floor.

Hold your fingers at shoulder pinnacle, attractive your deltoids.

Hold this option for a predetermined time (e.G., 20-30 seconds) even as making sure your shoulders stay solid.

3. Isometric Lateral Raise:

Stand tall with your feet shoulder-width aside and hands at your facets.

Raise your hands immediately out to the perimeters till they'll be parallel to the floor.

Engage your deltoid muscle companies as you maintain the raised role.

Hold this function for a predetermined time (e.G., 20-30 seconds) whilst keeping the peak of your hands.

four. Isometric External Rotation:

Stand along side your hands bent at 90 degrees and your elbows close to your components.

Rotate your forearms outward in opposition to resistance (e.G., resistance band or wall), appealing your shoulder muscular tissues.

Hold the outside rotation position for a predetermined time (e.G., 20-30 seconds) at the same time as keeping your elbows strong.

5. Isometric Shoulder Extension:

Stand together together along with your hands extended in advance at shoulder top.

Push your hands backward in competition to a stable floor, which include a wall or door body, engaging your posterior deltoids.

Hold this extended position for a predetermined time (e.G., 20-30 seconds) on the identical time as maintaining anxiety to your shoulders.

Important Considerations:

Maintain right posture and form in the direction of every isometric exercise to avoid straining your shoulders.

Breathe regularly at some point of the holds and avoid keeping your breath.

Begin with shorter maintain times and regularly growth the length as you assemble electricity and confidence.

Include a number of shoulder and deltoid wearing occasions to your regular higher frame workout routine for balanced muscle improvement.

Performing the ones isometric shoulder and deltoid bodily activities regularly can result in expanded shoulder strength, stepped forward posture, and reduced danger of shoulder-associated injuries. As with any exercise software, it's far important to tailor your everyday for your person fitness stage and dreams. If you've got had been given any gift shoulder issues or issues, don't forget searching out guidance from a health professional or healthcare company to ensure that your exercising plan aligns together together with your particular desires and competencies.

Back and Latissimus Dorsi Exercises

Strengthening the decrease again muscle groups, especially the latissimus dorsi or "lats," is crucial for keeping proper posture, improving pinnacle frame energy, and helping a wholesome backbone. Isometric sports activities sports offer an powerful manner to goal and have interaction the all over again muscular tissues, assisting to build power and stability. Below are a few isometric physical sports activities specially designed to art work the lower again and latissimus dorsi:

1. Wall Angels:

Stand collectively together with your decrease back in opposition to a wall and feet approximately a foot faraway from the wall.

Raise your fingers to shoulder diploma, keeping them in contact with the wall.

Slowly slide your hands upward, overhead, and then backpedal whilst preserving touch with the wall throughout.

Focus on attractive your decrease back muscle businesses, particularly the lats, ultimately of the motion.

Repeat for a predetermined time or amount of repetitions.

2. Isometric Pull-Up Hold:

Find a sturdy pull-up bar or robust a resistance band overhead to serve as an anchor.

Grab the bar or resistance band with an overhand grip, arms shoulder-width aside.

Lift your feet off the floor, helping your body weight collectively along with your fingers.

Hold yourself within the top characteristic of a pull-up collectively collectively with your chin above the bar, engaging your decrease returned muscular tissues, along with the lats.

Maintain this function for a predetermined time (e.G., 20-30 seconds) at the equal time as preserving your shoulders strong.

3. Isometric Row Hold:

Stand coping with an anchor element (e.G., a strong door cope with or resistance band secured to a wall).

Hold the resistance band with every arms and step back to create anxiety inside the band.

Position your palms immediately in the the the front of you, after which pull your elbows once more, squeezing your shoulder blades together.

Hold this feature together together with your elbows bent at approximately 90 levels, attractive your decrease once more muscle tissues and lats.

Maintain the row keep for a predetermined time (e.G., 20-30 seconds).

four. Plank with Row Hold:

Assume a plank characteristic with your forearms on the ground and your body in a instantly line from head to heels.

Hold a dumbbell or resistance band in a unmarried hand and preserve a strong plank feature.

Perform a row with the resource of pulling the weight up within the route of your chest, attractive your again muscle tissues, on the side of the lats.

Hold the top function of the row for a predetermined time, then transfer to the opportunity hand.

five. Isometric Superman Hold:

Lie face down at the ground collectively along with your hands prolonged overhead and legs at once.

Lift your fingers, chest, and legs off the floor, retaining a impartial neck function.

Squeeze your glutes and interact your lower returned muscle groups, which incorporates the lats, to maintain the prolonged feature.

Hold the Superman function for a predetermined time (e.G., 20-30 seconds).

Important Considerations:

Focus on attractive the over again muscle tissues, mainly the latissimus dorsi, during every isometric workout.

Keep your core engaged and maintain right shape to prevent stress and harm.

Breathe step by step and avoid preserving your breath in the end of the holds.

Begin with shorter maintain times and progressively growth the period as you boom once more energy.

Incorporating the ones isometric decrease lower back and latissimus dorsi carrying activities into your health regular can purpose extended returned electricity, improved posture, and more relevant fashionable pinnacle frame stability. As with any exercise utility, it is critical to pay interest on your body and regulate the wearing sports consistent with your fitness degree and dreams. If you have any gift decrease back problems or issues, recall searching out steerage from a fitness expert or healthcare provider to make sure that your workout plan aligns together with your particular goals and talents.

Arm and Bicep/Tricep Exercises

Strengthening the palms, consisting of the biceps and triceps, not fine complements your bodily appearance however also improves your everyday pinnacle body functionality. Isometric sports activities activities provide an effective manner to goal and interact the ones arm muscle tissue, promoting accelerated energy and muscular staying energy. Below are a few isometric physical video games specially designed to art work the fingers, biceps, and triceps:

Chapter 3: Isometric Exercises For Lower Body

Quadriceps and Hamstring Exercises

Isometric sporting sports for the decrease frame are alternatively effective for building strength, stability, and staying strength within the muscle organizations of the legs, in particular the quadriceps and hamstrings. These sporting sports activities provide a tough exercise without the need for complicated movements or device. Below are a few isometric sports specifically designed to goal the quadriceps and hamstrings:

1. Wall Sit:

Stand alongside facet your lower back in opposition to a wall and feet shoulder-width apart.

Slide your back off the wall until your knees are bent at a 90-diploma thoughts-set.

Hold this seated feature collectively along with your thighs parallel to the ground.

Engage your quadriceps in the course of the preserve.

Hold the position for a predetermined time (e.G., 20-30 seconds) at the equal time as keeping right shape and breathing step by step.

2. Static Lunge Hold:

Take a lunge stance with one foot in advance and the opposite foot once more.

Bend your knees to decrease your frame right right into a lunge role, ensuring every knees are at ninety-degree angles.

Hold the lunge feature, attractive the quadriceps of each legs.

Maintain an upright posture and keep for a predetermined time (e.G., 20-30 seconds) in advance than switching to the alternative leg.

three. Isometric Leg Extension:

Sit on a chair or bench at the side of your lower back proper away and feet flat on the floor.

Extend one leg directly out within the the the front of you, attractive your quadriceps.

Hold your leg inside the extended position for a predetermined time (e.G., 20-30 seconds).

Keep your returned immediately and middle engaged at some stage within the keep.

4. Isometric Bridge Hold:

Lie for your returned together with your knees bent and feet flat at the floor.

Lift your hips off the floor, growing a straight away line from your shoulders on your knees.

Squeeze your glutes and have interaction your hamstrings and quadriceps to preserve the bridge feature.

Hold the place for a predetermined time (e.G., 20-30 seconds).

5. Isometric Hamstring Curl:

Lie face down at the ground alongside facet your legs extended and your palms positioned below your hips for help.

Bend one knee to carry your heel inside the path of your glutes, appealing your hamstrings.

Hold the bent characteristic for a predetermined time (e.G., 20-30 seconds) before switching to the alternative leg.

Important Considerations:

Focus on engaging the focused muscle tissues (quadriceps or hamstrings) within the route of each isometric exercising.

Keep your center engaged and preserve right shape to save you pressure on your decrease again or knees.

Breathe regularly and keep away from protecting your breath at a few degree inside the holds.

Begin with shorter keep times and step by step growth the duration as you construct decrease frame energy.

Incorporating those isometric wearing sports for the quadriceps and hamstrings into your fitness recurring can reason accelerated lower body electricity, improved muscular patience, and higher not unusual decrease frame balance. As with any exercising utility, it's miles vital to take note of your frame and alter the sports in step with your health level and dreams. If you've got any present decrease frame troubles or worries, do not forget searching for guidance from a fitness professional or healthcare company to ensure that your workout plan aligns together with your particular dreams and abilties.

Gluteal and Hip Exercises

Strengthening the gluteal muscle corporations and hips is important for ordinary lower frame balance, mobility, and energy. Isometric wearing events provide an effective way to intention and engage the ones muscle companies, selling extended strength and versatility. Below are some isometric wearing sports activities especially designed to artwork the glutes and hips:

1. Glute Bridge Hold:

Lie on your decrease returned together together with your knees bent and feet flat on the ground, hip-width apart.

Press your heels into the floor and raise your hips off the floor, developing a immediately line out of your shoulders in your knees.

Squeeze your glutes and engage your middle to keep the bridge feature.

Hold this characteristic for a predetermined time (e.G., 20-30 seconds) on the identical time as keeping a strong bridge.

2. Isometric Clamshell Hold:

Lie to your component together along with your knees bent and stacked on top of every exceptional.

Keep your feet collectively and lift your top knee faraway from the bottom knee, developing tension in your glutes.

Hold the lifted function for a predetermined time (e.G., 20-30 seconds) earlier than switching to the possibility aspect.

3. Isometric Squat Hold:

Stand together with your ft shoulder-width apart or slightly wider, feet pointing slightly outward.

Lower your frame proper proper into a squat position, retaining your knees aligned collectively together with your toes.

Hold the squat feature together with your thighs parallel to the ground.

Engage your glutes and middle to preserve the squat maintain for a predetermined time (e.G., 20-30 seconds).

four. Isometric Hip Abduction:

Lie in your element together with your legs stacked on pinnacle of every special.

Lift your top leg far from the bottom leg, appealing your hip abductor muscle mass.

Hold the lifted position for a predetermined time (e.G., 20-30 seconds) earlier than switching to the opportunity thing.

five. Isometric Fire Hydrant Hold:

Begin on all fours together with your arms without delay below your shoulders and knees beneath your hips.

Lift one leg out to the element, bending your knee at a 90-diploma perspective (just like a dog lifting its leg).

Hold the lifted position together along with your knee bent, attractive your glutes.

Hold for a predetermined time (e.G., 20-30 seconds) in advance than switching to the opportunity leg.

Important Considerations:

Focus on attractive the centered muscle tissue (glutes and hips) sooner or later of every isometric exercise.

Keep your middle engaged and maintain proper form to save you strain to your lower again or knees.

Breathe little by little and keep away from maintaining your breath sooner or later of the holds.

Begin with shorter maintain times and regularly growth the duration as you construct gluteal and hip strength.

Incorporating those isometric sports activities activities for the glutes and hips into your fitness ordinary can result in stepped forward lower frame power, progressed hip balance, and stronger fashionable lower body functionality. As with any exercising software program, it's miles important to pay attention to your frame and alter the carrying sports consistent with your health level and goals. If you've got got had been given any present gluteal or hip issues or worries, take into account trying to find guidance from a fitness expert or healthcare employer to ensure that your workout plan aligns on the aspect of your particular wishes and abilties.

Calf and Shin Exercises

Strengthening the calf and shin muscle groups is crucial for decrease leg stability, balance, and widespread average overall performance in numerous bodily sports. Isometric sports offer an powerful way to purpose and have interaction those muscle mass, selling extended energy and resilience. Below are a few isometric physical activities especially designed to paintings the calves and shins:

1. Isometric Calf Raise Hold:

Stand collectively in conjunction with your feet hip-width apart close to a wall or strong aid for balance.

Raise your heels off the floor, lifting onto the balls of your feet.

Hold this position on the side of your calves engaged and heels expanded.

Maintain the calf decorate preserve for a predetermined time (e.G., 20-30 seconds) with out letting your heels contact the ground.

2. Wall Calf Stretch:

Stand dealing with a wall and location your palms at the wall at shoulder top.

Take a step once more with one foot and press the heel of that foot into the floor.

Keep your over again leg directly and your the front knee barely bent.

Hold this stretch with the another time calf muscle engaged for a predetermined time (e.G., 20-30 seconds).

Repeat the stretch on the opportunity leg.

three. Toe Tap Hold:

Sit on a chair or bench together with your ft flat at the ground.

Lift your feet off the floor, retaining your heels firmly planted.

Hold this characteristic along with your shins engaged and ft increased.

Maintain the toe faucet maintain for a predetermined time (e.G., 20-30 seconds).

4. Isometric Shin Push:

Sit on a chair together along with your knees bent at 90 stages and ft flat at the ground.

Place a resistance band or towel round your ft.

Press the balls of your feet in competition to the resistance band or towel, attractive your shin muscle groups.

Chapter 4: Core Strengthening Isometric Exercises

Abdominal and Oblique Exercises

A robust and stable middle is important for assisting your backbone, enhancing posture, and improving everyday frame electricity. Isometric physical sports offer an effective way to intention and engage the center muscle agencies, which incorporates the abdominals and obliques. Below are some isometric carrying events particularly designed to artwork the middle:

1. Plank Hold:

Start in a push-up function collectively together with your hands on the ground right now beneath your shoulders and ft on the ground.

Engage your middle and create a right now line out of your head to heels, fending off any sagging or arching to your yet again.

Hold the plank characteristic, collectively together with your abs and obliques engaged, for a predetermined time (e.G., 30-60 seconds).

2. Side Plank Hold:

Lie for your issue along side your elbow without delay below your shoulder and ft stacked on top of every different.

Lift your hips off the ground, developing a without delay line from your head to ft.

Engage your obliques and hold the side plank position for a predetermined time (e.G., 30-60 seconds) on each element.

3. Isometric Bicycle Crunch:

Lie for your lower again collectively in conjunction with your knees bent and fingers placed lightly in the back of your head.

Lift your shoulders off the ground and interact your middle.

Bring one knee toward your chest while concurrently rotating your torso to supply the opposite elbow in the path of the knee.

Hold this feature alongside facet your center engaged for a predetermined time (e.G., 20-30 seconds) earlier than switching to the alternative aspect.

four. Isometric Dead Bug:

Lie to your again in conjunction with your hands extended directly up toward the ceiling and knees bent at ninety ranges.

Lower one arm inside the again of your head and the other leg toward the floor, with out permitting them to touch the ground.

Engage your center to save you any movement for your returned or hips.

Hold this position for a predetermined time (e.G., 20-30 seconds) in advance than switching to the alternative facet.

five. Isometric Russian Twist:

Sit on the ground collectively together along with your knees bent and toes flat on the floor.

Lean another time slightly, keeping your lower returned directly and center engaged.

Hold your palms together in the front of your chest and twist your torso to at least one facet.

Engage your obliques and maintain the twist for a predetermined time (e.G., 20-30 seconds) earlier than switching to the possibility side.

Important Considerations:

Focus on engaging the center muscular tissues, which incorporates the abdominals and obliques, in the route of every isometric workout.

Maintain right form and avoid straining your neck or lower again at some degree within the holds.

Breathe step by step and keep away from defensive your breath in the course of the physical sports.

Begin with shorter hold times and little by little growth the length as you construct center power.

Incorporating those isometric center strengthening wearing sports into your fitness regular can bring about improved center balance, better belly and indirect power, and better regular body function. As with any exercising software, it is essential to pay attention for your frame and modify the wearing sports activities in keeping with your health degree and goals. If you have have been given any modern center or again issues or concerns, don't forget in search of guidance from a fitness expert or healthcare issuer to make sure that your exercising plan aligns collectively together with your unique needs and capabilities.

Lower Back Exercises

A sturdy and bendy decrease lower once more is critical for retaining a healthful spine, assisting proper posture, and preventing lower decrease once more ache. Isometric bodily video video games may be effective in targeting and engaging the muscle groups inside the decrease lower lower returned. Below are some isometric sporting occasions mainly designed to art work the decrease once more:

1. Superman Hold:

Lie face down on the floor collectively together with your arms extended overhead and legs without delay.

Lift your hands, chest, and legs off the floor concurrently, equal to the flying position of Superman.

Engage your lower again muscle organizations to preserve the improved role.

Hold the Superman function for a predetermined time (e.G., 20-30 seconds) even as keeping right alignment.

2. Bridge Hold:

Lie on your returned collectively along with your knees bent and feet flat at the floor, hip-width aside.

Lift your hips off the ground, developing a directly line out of your shoulders on your knees.

Squeeze your glutes and interact your decrease again to hold the bridge function.

Hold this function for a predetermined time (e.G., 20-30 seconds) at the equal time as keeping your center strong.

three. Bird-Dog Hold:

Start on all fours together with your fingers without delay beneath your shoulders and knees under your hips.

Extend your right arm uncomplicated while simultaneously extending your left leg right away back.

Engage your lower lower returned and middle to preserve this prolonged function.

Hold the Bird-Dog role for a predetermined time (e.G., 20-30 seconds) earlier than switching to the opposite aspect.

4. Dead Bug Hold:

Lie to your lower back together with your palms prolonged in the direction of the ceiling and knees bent at ninety ranges.

Lower one arm in the once more of your head and the other leg closer to the floor, with out letting them contact the floor.

Engage your decrease returned to prevent any motion in your lower back or hips.

Hold this role for a predetermined time (e.G., 20-30 seconds) earlier than switching to the alternative issue.

5. Wall Plank Hold:

Stand going via a wall and place your palms on the wall at shoulder height.

Walk your toes once more, leaning your frame into the wall at a mild mindset.

Engage your decrease again and center to hold a directly line out of your head to heels.

Hold the wall plank role for a predetermined time (e.G., 20-30 seconds) on the same time as focusing on your lower lower again muscular tissues.

Important Considerations:

Focus on attractive the decrease once more muscle mass at some point of each isometric exercising to avoid straining the backbone.

Maintain right shape and alignment inside the direction of the holds to prevent any undue pressure at the decrease lower returned.

Breathe step by step and avoid protecting your breath inside the path of the physical games.

Begin with shorter preserve times and often boom the length as you build lower again power and persistence.

Incorporating the ones isometric decrease once more carrying events into your fitness normal can result in superior decrease another time electricity, extra awesome spinal help, and decreased chance of decrease once more ache. As with any exercise utility, it's far essential to concentrate on your frame and regulate the sports in step with your fitness degree and desires. If you have any gift decrease decrease again problems or worries, bear in mind searching for guidance from a fitness expert or healthcare provider to ensure that your exercising plan aligns alongside aspect your precise desires and skills.

Chapter 5: Total Body Isometric Workout Routines

Beginner's Full-Body Routine

Isometric carrying events provide a remarkable entire-body workout that can be tailor-made to healthful human beings of all fitness ranges, inclusive of novices. This everyday objectives essential muscle businesses even as improving ordinary strength and balance. Perform each workout for the encouraged length or big fashion of repetitions, and remember to maintain proper shape and have interaction the focused muscle tissue within the route of each hold. As a beginner, begin with shorter maintain times and steadily increase the period as you emerge as extra snug with the sports activities.

Warm-up:

Before beginning the habitual, spend 5-10 minutes appearing dynamic stretches or mild cardiovascular sports activities to heat up your muscle mass.

1. Isometric wall sit down:

Stand at the side of your lower back in opposition to a wall and slide down until your knees are bent at a ninety-diploma attitude.

Engage your quadriceps and preserve the wall sit down feature for 20-30 seconds.

2. Isometric Push-up Hold:

Assume a plank position together with your palms on the floor straight away beneath your shoulders and feet on the floor.

Lower your body down until your chest is a few inches from the floor.

Hold the mid-push-up feature alongside side your fingers barely bent for 20-30 seconds.

three. Isometric Bodyweight Squat:

Stand on the aspect of your toes shoulder-width aside and feet barely grew to turn out to be outward.

Lower your body right right into a squat feature, knees bent at a 90-diploma thoughts-set.

Hold the squat characteristic together along with your thighs parallel to the floor for 20-30 seconds.

4. Isometric Plank Hold:

Lie for your stomach and raise your body off the floor, supporting your self for your forearms and toes.

Keep your frame in a at once line from head to heels and hold the plank function for 20-30 seconds.

five. Isometric Superman Hold:

Lie on your belly together along with your arms prolonged overhead and legs right away.

Lift your arms, chest, and legs off the floor simultaneously.

Engage your decrease lower again and keep the Superman function for 20-30 seconds.

6. Isometric Glute Bridge Hold:

Lie to your decrease returned together with your knees bent and ft flat on the floor.

Lift your hips off the ground, developing a immediately line from your shoulders to knees.

Squeeze your glutes and preserve the glute bridge feature for 20-30 seconds.

7. Isometric Bicep Curl Hold:

Stand together in conjunction with your toes shoulder-width apart and hold dumbbells at your aspects with an underhand grip.

Curl the weights inside the course of your shoulders, enticing your biceps.

Hold the reduced in size position collectively with your elbows bent at approximately ninety stages for 20-30 seconds.

eight. Isometric Shoulder Press Hold:

Stand tall together together with your ft shoulder-width apart and dumbbells at shoulder top, hands managing forward.

Press the dumbbells overhead, attractive your shoulder muscle tissues.

Hold the overhead role on the facet of your palms honestly extended for 20-30 seconds.

Cool Down:

Finish the ordinary with 5-10 mins of static stretching, specializing in principal muscle organizations.

Important Considerations:

Perform this ordinary 2-3 times in line with week with at least one day of relaxation among periods.

Focus on proper shape and interact the centered muscle tissues for the period of each isometric exercising.

Begin with shorter preserve instances and regularly increase the length as you benefit power and self belief.

Consult with a fitness expert or healthcare company when you have any pre-present day fitness situations or problems.

The novice's complete-body isometric routine offers an extraordinary basis for building electricity, balance, and staying power in the direction of the whole frame. As you improvement, enjoy loose to feature more repetitions or increase the hold instances to undertaking yourself in addition. Remember that consistency and staying power are key to achieving your health dreams.

Intermediate Total Body Routine

Congratulations on advancing to the intermediate degree! This famous body isometric regular is designed to take your strength and stability to the subsequent stage. It objectives important muscle agencies and consists of greater difficult bodily sports activities. Perform each workout for the encouraged length or repetitions, focusing on proper form and appealing the targeted muscle groups within the path of every preserve.

Warm-up:

Begin with five-10 minutes of dynamic stretches and mild cardiovascular wearing sports to heat up your muscles.

1. Isometric Bulgarian Split Squat:

Stand coping with a ways from a knee-immoderate platform or bench.

Place one foot on the platform in the back of you and reduce right into a lunge role, the front knee bent at a 90-diploma mind-set.

Hold the split squat function collectively along with your once more foot extended for 30 seconds on every leg.

2. Isometric Push-up with Knee Tap:

Assume a plank characteristic collectively collectively with your palms at the floor at once underneath your shoulders and ft at the ground.

Lower your body down till your chest is a few inches from the ground.

Hold the mid-push-up feature even as tapping your right knee in your proper elbow and then your left knee on your left elbow. Alternate faucets for 30 seconds.

three. Isometric Squat Hold with Calf Raises:

Stand along side your toes shoulder-width aside.

Lower your frame right right into a squat characteristic, knees bent at a 90-diploma mindset.

Hold the squat feature for 30 seconds after which upward thrust onto the balls of your toes to perform calf will increase for 15 seconds.

4. Isometric Plank with Shoulder Taps:

Assume a plank characteristic collectively collectively along with your hands at the ground right now beneath your shoulders and toes slightly wider than hip-width apart.

Engage your middle and glutes to stabilize your frame.

Tap your proper hand for your left shoulder and then your left hand on your proper shoulder. Alternate faucets for 30 seconds.

5. Isometric Superman with Arm and Leg Lift:

Lie on your belly together along with your hands extended overhead and legs proper away.

Lift your arms, chest, and legs off the ground concurrently.

Engage your lower lower back and lift your right arm and left leg higher whilst maintaining the Superman feature for 15 seconds. Switch aspects and keep for each special 15 seconds.

6. Isometric Bridge with Marching:

Lie in your lower returned at the side of your knees bent and ft flat at the ground.

Lift your hips off the floor, growing a straight away line out of your shoulders to knees.

Engage your glutes and center at the same time as lifting one foot off the ground, bringing your knee within the direction of your chest. Alternate legs for 30 seconds.

Stand together along with your ft shoulder-width apart and maintain dumbbells at your sides with a unbiased grip (fingers going via each one-of-a-type).

7. Isometric Hammer Curl and Shoulder Press:

Perform a hammer curl through curling the weights inside the route of your shoulders.

Then, press the dumbbells overhead, attractive your shoulders.

Hold the overhead function for 10 seconds earlier than returning to the begin function.

eight. Isometric Plank Walkouts:

Start in a plank function collectively collectively with your arms on the ground at once under your shoulders and toes at the floor.

Walk your hands earlier, one at a time, as a ways as you can even as retaining a sturdy plank function.

Then, walk your fingers once more to the start function, regardless of the truth that maintaining proper shape. Repeat for 30 seconds.

Cool Down:

Finish the ordinary with five-10 minutes of static stretching, concentrated on primary muscle businesses.

Important Considerations:

Perform this intermediate ordinary 2-3 times in step with week with at the least someday of relaxation amongst training.

Focus on attractive the centered muscle tissue in the end of every isometric workout and maintaining right form at some point of.

Challenge your self with longer maintain times and additional repetitions as you development.

If you have any pre-present fitness conditions or concerns, are looking for recommendation from a health expert or healthcare provider.

The intermediate considerable body isometric recurring will help you hold constructing power, balance, and staying electricity on the equal time as retaining your workout workouts hard and worthwhile. Remember to pay interest to your body, and stay devoted on your fitness adventure for optimum notable effects.

Advanced Full-Body Challenge

Congratulations on achieving the advanced degree! This full-frame isometric assignment is designed to push your energy, stability, and staying energy to the limit. It includes immoderate and annoying physical video games that concentrate on multiple muscle businesses concurrently. Perform each exercising for the recommended period or repetitions, specializing in maintaining right form and appealing the centered muscle tissues in some unspecified time inside the destiny of every maintain.

Warm-up:

Begin with 5-10 mins of dynamic stretches and light cardiovascular physical activities to thoroughly warmth up your muscle tissue.

1. Isometric Pistol Squat:

Stand on one leg with the alternative leg extended immediately out in front of you.

Slowly lower your self right right into a single-leg squat characteristic, keeping your lower decrease back without delay and chest lifted.

Hold the pistol squat function along side your prolonged leg parallel to the floor for 30 seconds on every leg.

2. Isometric Push-up to T-Plank:

Assume a plank feature on the aspect of your fingers at the ground immediately below your shoulders and toes at the ground.

Lower your frame down till your chest is a few inches from the floor.

Press returned as lots because the plank function and raise one arm off the floor, extending it right away as an entire lot as shape a T shape alongside facet your body.

Hold the T-plank function for some seconds in advance than returning to the beginning function. Alternate elements for 30 seconds.

three. Isometric Sumo Squat Hold with Calf Raises:

Stand alongside facet your ft wider than shoulder-width apart and feet grew to come to be barely outward.

Lower your frame right into a sumo squat function, knees bent and thighs parallel to the floor.

Hold the sumo squat function for 30 seconds and then upward push onto the balls of your ft to perform calf increases for 15 seconds.

four. Isometric Plank with Alternating Leg Lift:

Assume a plank characteristic collectively together with your hands at the floor right now beneath your shoulders and feet slightly wider than hip-width aside.

Engage your middle and glutes to stabilize your frame.

Lift one leg a few inches off the floor, preserve for a few seconds, after which transfer legs. Continue alternating for 30 seconds.

5. Isometric Superman with Arm and Leg Extension:

Lie to your stomach together along with your fingers prolonged overhead and legs right away.

Lift your palms, chest, and legs off the floor concurrently.

Engage your lower again and raise your right arm and left leg better at the equal time as shielding the Superman characteristic for 15 seconds. Switch factors and maintain for some other 15 seconds.

6. Isometric Bridge with Leg Curl:

Lie for your once more collectively along with your knees bent and feet flat on the floor.

Lift your hips off the ground, growing a at once line from your shoulders to knees.

Engage your glutes and center even as curling one leg inside the direction of your glutes. Alternate legs for 30 seconds.

7. Isometric Tricep Dip Hold:

Sit on the point of a sturdy chair or bench along with your palms gripping the threshold beside your hips.

Walk your feet earlier and lift your hips off the chair.

Lower your frame down right into a dip role and preserve the isometric tricep dip for 30 seconds.

8. Isometric Plank with Alternating Arm and Leg Reach:

Assume a plank function collectively with your hands on the ground right away underneath your shoulders and ft barely wider than hip-width apart.

Engage your middle and glutes to stabilize your frame.

Lift your proper arm and left leg off the ground and reap them ahead and backward, respectively.

Return to the plank role and repeat on the opportunity issue. Continue alternating for 30 seconds.

Cool Down:

Finish the mission with 5-10 minutes of static stretching, specializing in number one muscle companies.

Important Considerations:

Perform this advanced entire-frame isometric undertaking 2-3 times in step with week, giving your self sufficient relaxation amongst training.

Focus on retaining right shape and attractive the focused muscle groups all through each exercising.

Challenge your self with longer hold instances and similarly repetitions to maximize the intensity.

If you've got any pre-gift health situations or issues, talk with a health professional or healthcare employer.

The superior whole-frame isometric assignment will push your limits and take your health to new heights. Stay committed, concentrate in your body, and revel in the pleasure of conquering this rigorous workout habitual. Remember to have a excellent time your improvement and hold difficult yourself for your fitness adventure.

Chapter 6: Training Methods

Isometric Supersets and Circuits

Isometric sporting occasions can be covered with distinct education methods to create quite powerful and dynamic workout workouts. Two well-known techniques to mix isometrics with one in every of a kind carrying events are via isometric supersets and isometric circuits. These strategies add variety, intensity, and project on your exercising sporting activities while focused on high-quality muscle companies for complete training.

1. Isometric Supersets:

Isometric supersets comprise pairing an isometric exercise with a conventional dynamic exercising targeting the same or opposing muscle agencies. The mixture lets in you to artwork on every power and balance at the same time as improving muscle activation. Here's the manner to contain isometric supersets into your training:

Example:

Isometric Squat Hold (Isometric Exercise): Hold a squat characteristic for 30 seconds.

Barbell Back Squat (Dynamic Exercise): Perform 8-10 reps of barbell decrease lower back squats immediately after the isometric preserve.

Instructions:

1. Complete the isometric squat keep, focusing on attractive your quadriceps and glutes in the route of the maintain.

2. Immediately transition to the barbell yet again squats, retaining right shape and the usage of a hard weight.

three. Rest for 60-90 seconds in advance than repeating the superset for the desired range of gadgets.

2. Isometric Circuits:

Isometric circuits incorporate performing a sequence of isometric wearing sports consecutively, focused on special muscle groups. This method demanding situations your muscular persistence and cardiovascular device at the same time as improving normal body strength. Here's an example of an isometric circuit:

Example:

Perform each exercise for 30 seconds with out a relaxation in amongst:

Plank Hold: Assume a plank position, enticing your center and retaining a straight away line from head to heels.

Wall Sit: Lean in opposition to a wall together together with your knees bent at a 90-degree mind-set, enticing your quadriceps.

Isometric Push-up Hold: Lower your frame to the midpoint of a push-up and hold the location at the side of your hands slightly bent.

Instructions:

1. Start with the plank hold for 30 seconds, focusing on middle stability and proper alignment.

2. Immediately transition to the wall sit down down, retaining the squat function for 30 seconds, concentrated on your quadriceps.

3. Move proper away to the isometric push-up keep, appealing your chest and triceps for each other 30 seconds.

four. After completing all three sporting sports, rest for 60 seconds, and then repeat the circuit for the favored amount of rounds.

Important Considerations:

Ensure right shape and have interaction the targeted muscle companies for the duration of every isometric exercising in the superset or circuit.

Rest amongst supersets or circuits to permit for properly enough healing before beginning the following spherical.

Adjust the length or intensity of the isometric bodily sports to fit your fitness degree and desires.

Incorporate isometric supersets and circuits into your training normal once or twice in step with week to avoid overtraining.

Combining isometrics with one of a kind training strategies gives versatility and task for your workout workouts. These techniques effectively engage first rate muscle groups, beautify muscular patience, and make contributions to traditional electricity earnings. As with any exercising routine, pay interest for your body, and alter the sports as desired to fit your fitness level and skills. Additionally, consulting with a fitness professional can offer customized steerage to optimize your education experience.

Incorporating Isometrics into Weight Training

Isometric sporting sports may be seamlessly covered into your weight education ordinary, enhancing muscle activation, electricity earnings, and average workout effectiveness. By incorporating isometrics, you upload a totally precise length on your weight education, attractive muscle agencies in every other way than traditional dynamic actions. Here are several methods to embody isometrics into your weight schooling habitual:

1. Isometric Holds:

Integrate isometric holds at unique points in some unspecified time within the destiny of weightlifting carrying events to aim precise muscle corporations and growth time below anxiety. Hold a weight at a tremendous feature for a predetermined period to challenge your muscle agencies similarly.

Example:

During a barbell bench press, pause and preserve the barbell on the midpoint (at the same time as your palms are bent at ninety degrees) for 5-10 seconds earlier than finishing the whole repetition.

2. Isometric Contractions with Weights:

Combine isometric contractions with weightlifting sporting occasions to spark off greater muscle fibers and decorate electricity and balance.

Example:

Perform a bicep curl with dumbbells and pause halfway thru the curl, maintaining the weights at a ninety-diploma angle for five-10 seconds earlier than finishing the curl.

three. Isometric Supersets:

Create supersets by means of the usage of way of pairing an isometric exercising with a weight schooling exercise focused at the equal muscle organization or an opposing one. This mixture stimulates extra muscle activation and builds energy.

Example:

Pair a **plank preserve** (isometric exercising) with **dumbbell rows** (dynamic exercising). Perform a 30-2d plank preserve, discovered proper away via a hard and fast of 8-10 dumbbell rows.

4. Isometric Eccentric Training:

Incorporate isometric contractions during the eccentric (reducing) section of weightlifting carrying occasions. This approach will boom muscle anxiety and might decorate power earnings.

Example:

During a barbell squat, decrease into the squat feature slowly and pause midway down for an isometric maintain earlier than completing the squat.

five. Isometric Core Engagement:

Engage your middle isometrically in the direction of diverse weight schooling carrying activities to stabilize your backbone and decorate standard strength.

Example:

During a **barbell shoulder press**, interact your middle muscle mass to hold proper posture and prevent excessive arching in your lower decrease again.

6. Isometric Finishing Holds:

Incorporate isometric finishing holds on the end of your weight schooling units to assignment your muscle organizations to their limits.

Example:

After finishing a hard and fast of **dumbbell lunges**, preserve the lunge role for a further 10-15 seconds earlier than switching to the alternative leg.

Important Considerations:

Prioritize right shape and method in the course of every the isometric and weight education sports activities.

Start with shorter maintain instances and steadily boom the period as you grow to be more comfortable with isometrics.

Avoid retaining your breath in the course of isometric contractions; keep steady respiratory in the course of.

Listen in your body and adjust the intensity and length of isometrics primarily based completely in your fitness diploma and goals.

Incorporating isometrics into your weight education regular can be an powerful technique for building electricity, growing muscle activation, and diversifying your sporting activities. Whether you are a amateur or an expert lifter, isometric carrying events offer precious advantages that supplement your present weight training software program. Remember to venture yourself steadily, and speak over with a health professional in case you're unsure about proper execution or modifications on your character wishes.

Isometrics for Endurance and Flexibility

Isometric physical games are often related to building energy and stability, however they also can play a large characteristic in improving patience and flexibility. By incorporating specific isometric strategies into your schooling habitual, you could enhance your stamina, increase your variety of motion, and increase more flexibility. Here's the way to use isometrics for staying electricity and flexibility training:

1. Isometric Endurance Training:

Isometric physical video games may be changed to recognition on developing muscular staying power, allowing you to maintain positions for longer intervals. Endurance-targeted isometrics interact sluggish-twitch muscle fibers, which can be accountable for sustained contractions over time. Here's the way to apply isometric physical video games for patience schooling:

Example: Isometric Wall Sit for Endurance:

Stand collectively at the side of your lower back in competition to a wall and slide down till your knees are bent at a ninety-degree mind-set, simulating a seated role.

Engage your quadriceps and hold the wall sit feature for so long as viable, aiming for 60 seconds or greater.

Gradually artwork inside the direction of increasing the keep time as your staying energy improves.

2. Isometric Flexibility Training:

Isometrics additionally may be carried out to decorate flexibility with the aid of using attractive muscle mass on the end in their form of motion. This technique is referred to as isometric stretching or PNF (Proprioceptive Neuromuscular Facilitation) stretching. By contracting and relaxing the muscular tissues in the course of stretching, you can accumulate greater income in flexibility. Here's a way to use isometric bodily sports for flexibility education:

Example: Isometric Hamstring Stretch:

Sit at the floor with one leg prolonged right away within the the front of you and the opposite leg bent at the knee.

Lean in advance from the hips to reap for your ft at the prolonged leg.

As you enjoy the stretch, lightly push your foot in opposition to the ground (isometric contraction) for five-10 seconds.

Relax the rush and deepen the stretch for another 10-15 seconds.

Repeat the isometric contraction and stretch one or extra instances.

three. Isometric Combination for Endurance and Flexibility:

Combining staying energy and versatility education can be completed via the use of incorporating isometric stretches into your regular. This approach allows you construct flexibility even as enhancing the potential to hold a stretched feature for longer intervals. Here's an instance:

Example: Isometric Quad Stretch for Endurance and Flexibility:

Stand collectively in conjunction with your feet together, and bring one heel within the path of your glutes to stretch your quadriceps.

Gently pull your ankle towards your glutes on the aspect of your hand on the same time as contracting your quadriceps (pushing your foot into your hand) for five-10 seconds.

Release the contraction slightly and deepen the stretch for 10-15 seconds.

Repeat the isometric contraction and stretch one or two greater instances.

Important Considerations:

Warm-up in advance than challenge isometric staying strength and versatility education to put together your muscular tissues for the bodily video video games.

Incorporate isometric physical games for staying power and versatility 2-three instances steady with week for max useful outcomes.

Listen in your frame and avoid pushing your self to the factor of pain in the route of stretching or staying power holds.

Combine isometric physical sports with dynamic stretches and conventional endurance wearing sports for a well-rounded schooling ordinary.

By adding isometric bodily games to your staying power and versatility training, you could decorate your athletic common performance, prevent injuries, and experience advanced useful movement. Remember to exercising staying power and consistency as improvement can also take time, especially at the same time as operating on flexibility gains. If you're new to those schooling techniques or have particular flexibility worries, recollect looking for steerage from a fitness professional or an authorized flexibility train to make certain secure and powerful education.

Chapter 7: Progression And Tracking Your Isometric Training

Setting Goals and Measuring Progress

Effectively progressing on your isometric education adventure includes setting easy dreams and monitoring your achievements over time. By setting up possible goals and tracking your development, you can live encouraged and make knowledgeable modifications for your exercising normal. Here's the way to set goals and degree your improvements in isometric training:

1. Establish Clear Goals:

Start via defining particular and sensible desires to your isometric education. Consider what you want to gain, whether it's miles extended energy, advanced endurance, greater flexibility, or focused on particular muscle companies. Having clean desires will supply your schooling cause and course.

Example Goals:

Increase plank preserve time from 30 seconds to 60 seconds in 4 weeks.

Achieve a ninety-degree wall sit down feature for forty five seconds within three months.

Enhance hamstring flexibility through reaching toes with out issues inside two months.

2. Record Baseline Measurements:

Before setting out your isometric training utility, file baseline measurements for the bodily video video games you recommend to awareness on. This will serve as a place to start to compare your development. Note down the length of holds, the form of repetitions, or the sort of motion for flexibility carrying sports.

three. Utilize Progression Techniques:

To keep difficult your muscle groups and making income, encompass improvement techniques into your isometric training. Gradually increase maintain times, add repetitions, or deepen stretches as you turn out to be more cushty with the sporting activities.

Example Progression Techniques:

Add 5 seconds on your plank hold each week until you obtain your motive time.

Increase the style of gadgets for isometric carrying sports from three to 4 over a month.

Gradually decrease the assist whilst acting isometric stretches to deepen the stretch.

four. Track Your Workouts:

Maintain a exercise log to tune every isometric exercise session. Record the bodily video video games performed, the duration of holds or repetitions, and any exquisite observations. Tracking your exercising sporting events allows you to recognize patterns and affirm your development objectively.

5. Regular Assessments:

Schedule everyday checks, along with each four weeks, to assess your development in the course of your dreams. Revisit the baseline measurements and evaluate them in conjunction with your current talents. Celebrate your achievements and make vital adjustments on your schooling plan.

6. Listen to Your Body:

While putting and pursuing dreams is vital, it's miles similarly important to pay hobby on your frame and avoid pushing yourself to the component of harm or immoderate strain. Always prioritize right form and technique in some unspecified time in the future of isometric carrying activities.

7. Modify Goals as Needed:

As you progress for your isometric education, your desires can also need to be modified or advanced. Adjust your desires to residence new worrying conditions or aspirations, retaining your training clean and attractive.

eight. Celebrate Milestones:

Take the time to have fun your milestones and accomplishments. Whether it's miles retaining a tough function for longer or undertaking greater flexibility, acknowledging your development will preserve you stimulated and dedicated for your training.

Important Considerations:

Set realistic and feasible dreams that align together along with your present day fitness degree and competencies.

Stay ordinary in conjunction with your isometric training, adhering to a normal time desk.

Stay affected character and understand that improvement may additionally additionally additionally range from man or woman to person.

Seek recommendation from health experts if you need steering on right progression techniques or changes to your schooling plan.

By putting dreams, monitoring improvement, and constantly tough yourself, you can make consistent enhancements for your isometric training. Regularly assessing your achievements and adjusting your education plan will bring about extra enhancements in power, endurance, and flexibility. Remember that every leap forward is a testomony in your electricity of thoughts and hard artwork, and your journey in isometric schooling is a private, rewarding revel in.

Gradual Intensity Increase

Gradual intensity increase is a key principle in isometric training that includes regularly difficult your muscle companies through the years. By regularly developing the problem of your isometric carrying sports activities, you may generally stimulate muscle boom, electricity gains, and common development in basic overall performance. This method permits save you plateaus and decreases the chance of harm. Here's the way to apply gradual depth boom in your isometric education:

1. Start at an Appropriate Level:

Begin your isometric training at a diploma that suits your modern health and power. Focus on reading proper shape and technique in advance than advancing to extra hard versions.

2. Lengthen Hold Times:

As you become cushty with an isometric exercising, boom the period of your holds. Gradually upload some seconds each week or training consultation to increase the time under tension.

Example:

If you can keep a plank role for 30 seconds, purpose to boom it to 35 seconds in the following week and preserve progressing till you attain your aim keep time.

3. Increase Repetitions or Sets:

Another way to progressively accentuate your isometric schooling is through growing the range of repetitions or units completed subsequently of each exercising.

Example:

If you perform three gadgets of wall sits for 30 seconds each, try growing to four sets or maintaining every set for 35 seconds.

four. Incorporate Advanced Variations:

Once you've got mastered the number one isometric sports activities, preserve in mind incorporating superior versions or more hard positions to similarly undertaking your muscle tissues.

Example:

For the plank workout, development to acting plank variations along with the plank with shoulder faucets or the plank with leg lifts.

five. Add External Resistance:

In a few isometric bodily video video games, you can upload out of doors resistance to increase the trouble. This need to incorporate using resistance bands, weights, or different device.

Example:

For the glute bridge exercising, vicinity a resistance band around your thighs and press in the direction of the band throughout the keep for introduced resistance.

6. Increase Range of Motion:

In isometric stretches, frequently boom the kind of motion all through the maintain to deepen the stretch and decorate flexibility.

Example:

When acting a hamstring stretch, gently try to reap in the direction of your feet in the route of the isometric keep.

7. Listen to Your Body:

Pay interest to how your body responds to the gradual depth growth. If you revel in immoderate pain or discomfort, regulate the improvement and permit more time for recuperation.

8. Incorporate Rest Days:

Ensure you have got true enough rest days amongst severe isometric workout workouts to permit your muscle tissues to get better and adapt.

nine. Celebrate Achievements:

Acknowledge and have fun your improvement as you bought your dreams and gain new stages of intensity. Positive reinforcement will hold you stimulated and committed to your education journey.

Important Considerations:

Gradual depth increase is vital to save you overtraining and decrease the danger of accidents.

Prioritize proper form and method at some point of each exercise to ensure protection and effectiveness.

Progress at a pace that is cushty for you, and be affected character collectively along with your body's natural version machine.

By imposing gradual intensity boom into your isometric education, you may continuously venture your muscular tissues, decorate your overall performance, and attain your fitness goals. Remember that ordinary improvement is greater sustainable ultimately, and consistency is high to making huge strides to your isometric training adventure.

Avoiding Plateaus and Overtraining

Plateaus and overtraining can avoid your improvement and result in frustration in isometric education. However, with proper making plans and cognizance, you can avoid the ones obstacles and keep making steady improvements. Here are vital techniques to avoid plateaus and overtraining on your isometric training:

1. Progressive Overload:

Incorporate the precept of modern overload, which entails often growing the intensity of your isometric sports activities sports through the years. As your muscle agencies adapt to the modern workload, upload extra challenge by means of using manner of extending preserve times, growing repetitions, or incorporating advanced variations.

2. Vary Your Routine:

Avoid doing the equal isometric sports each workout. Incorporate variety by way of collectively with precise sports activities and versions that concentrate on numerous muscle agencies. Varying your habitual keeps your muscle corporations engaged and stops version to unique moves.

3. Implement Periodization:

Utilize periodization to your schooling plan, which incorporates dividing your schooling into super stages with numerous intensities and dreams. Periodization lets in for installed development and restoration, decreasing the hazard of overtraining and maintaining your sporting activities sparkling.

four. Listen to Your Body:

Pay close to interest to how your body responds to your isometric education. If you sense excessively fatigued, revel in persistent ache, or look at a decline in overall performance, it may be a sign of overtraining. Listen on your body's signals and regulate your training as needed.

Chapter 8: Common Mistakes And How To Avoid Them

Technique Errors and Corrections

Maintaining right method is essential in isometric schooling to make certain safety, effectiveness, and maximum efficient effects. However, severa not unusual mistakes can avert improvement and growth the threat of harm. By being aware of those errors and imposing appropriate corrections, you can beautify the best of your isometric physical video video games. Here are some commonplace errors and a way to avoid them:

1. Poor Body Alignment:

Mistake: Allowing your frame to fall apart or arch during isometric physical video games can location pointless strain on your joints and decrease the effectiveness of the workout.

Correction: Focus on retaining a independent backbone and proper body alignment at some point of every isometric preserve. Engage your center muscles to stabilize your spine and avoid excessive arching or rounding of the decrease back.

2. Holding Your Breath:

Mistake: Holding your breath inside the course of isometric contractions can boom intra-stomach pressure, most important to dizziness and reduced oxygen supply in your muscle mass.

Correction: Breathe frequently and deeply for the length of each isometric keep. Inhale thru your nose in advance than starting the contraction, and exhale slowly through your mouth as you preserve the place. Maintaining right respiration complements fashionable wellknown overall performance and prevents unnecessary tension.

three. Overstraining and Jerking Movements:

Correction: Perform isometric bodily games with managed and easy actions. Avoid sudden jerks or bouncing, and attention on constant contractions and holds to engage the focused muscle groups correctly.

four. Neglecting Warm-up and Cool-down:

Mistake: Skipping heat-up physical games can boom the risk of harm, even as neglecting the cool-down segment can result in muscle tightness and ache.

Correction: Prioritize a dynamic warm temperature-up, in conjunction with mild aerobic, dynamic stretches, and mobility sporting events, to put together your muscle businesses for the isometric workout. After the consultation, carry out static stretches to sell muscle flexibility and resource in restoration.

5. Ignoring Proper Progression:

Mistake: Rushing into superior isometric physical video video games without studying the fundamentals can result in horrible shape and inadequate muscle engagement.

Correction: Start with foundational isometric bodily games, making sure you have were given right shape and stability. Gradually development to extra difficult variations as you advantage energy and self perception in your abilities.

6. Neglecting Core Engagement:

Mistake: Failing to have interaction your center in the course of isometric physical sports can compromise stability and save you muscle activation.

Correction: Focus on keeping middle activation for the duration of each isometric preserve. A robust center not best protects your spine however moreover complements the effectiveness of the workout.

7. Not Adjusting Equipment Properly:

Mistake: Improperly adjusting system, inclusive of resistance bands or weights, can cause suboptimal effects or possibly damage.

Correction: Ensure that any device used to your isometric training is adjusted to the right tension or load for your fitness degree. Follow right protection pointers and instructions furnished by using the usage of the use of the tool manufacturer.

8. Overtraining Specific Muscle Groups:

Mistake: Focusing absolutely on one muscle business enterprise with out giving sufficient time for rest and recuperation can motive muscle imbalances and overuse accidents.

Correction: Design a properly-rounded isometric education recurring that goals diverse muscle organizations and contains rest days among intense durations. Balanced education permits promote easy power and stops overtraining.

Important Considerations:

Seek steering from a health expert to research right form and method for isometric bodily sports, specially in case you're new to this form of schooling.

Perform isometric sporting sports within a pain-free shape of movement to keep away from damage.

Be aware of your body's barriers and keep away from pushing your self to the aspect of discomfort or pain.

By avoiding those common mistakes and that specialize in right approach, you could make the maximum of your isometric training and improvement correctly and efficaciously. Regularly test your form, be affected character at the side of your progress, and bear in thoughts that steady, aware education yields the extremely good consequences in the end.

Injury Prevention Tips

Incorporating damage prevention techniques into your isometric education everyday is essential for ensuring a secure and a achievement health journey. By following those pointers, you can reduce the risk of injuries and hold your body wholesome and robust inside the path of your isometric sporting events:

1. Warm-up Properly:

Always start your isometric schooling periods with a dynamic warmth-up. Engage in mild cardiovascular bodily sports like running, jumping jacks, or cycling to increase blood glide to your muscle agencies. Follow this with dynamic stretches to put together your body for the upcoming exercise.

2. Focus on Proper Form:

Maintain proper shape at some point of every isometric exercising. Incorrect shape can reason vain strain on muscle groups and joints, developing the threat of damage. If you're unsure about the first-rate approach, are attempting to find guidance from a fitness expert.

three. Start Slow and Progress Gradually:

Begin your isometric training on the right diploma on your cutting-edge fitness degree and often growth the intensity over the years. Avoid pushing yourself too hard too soon, as this can bring about overuse injuries and muscle lines.

4. Use Adequate Support:

When acting isometric sports activities that comprise balancing on one leg or arm, use a solid ground or help to help in maintaining balance and stability. This will help prevent falls and capacity injuries.

five. Avoid Overtraining:

Allow enough time for rest and healing among excessive isometric workout routines. Overtraining can result in muscle fatigue, improved damage hazard, and decreased average performance. Listen in your frame and deliver it the time it needs to get higher.

6. Incorporate Cross-Training:

Include loads of sports activities sports for your fitness recurring to prevent overuse injuries and muscle imbalances. Crossschooling with particular modalities which include cardiovascular sporting events, strength training, and flexibility physical activities can promote famous fitness and decrease the stress on unique muscle groups.

7. Listen to Your Body:

Pay hobby to any signs and symptoms of soreness, pain, or fatigue all through your isometric schooling. If you enjoy pain, prevent the workout immediately and are searching for professional advice if wished.

eight. Stay Hydrated:

Drink hundreds of water earlier than, in the course of, and after your physical games to stay hydrated. Proper hydration lets in premier muscle characteristic and aids in recuperation.

9. Stretch After Workouts:

Perform static stretches after your isometric training consultation to decorate flexibility and decrease muscle tightness. Focus on predominant muscle groups used in the route of the workout.

10. Maintain a Balanced Diet:

Fuel your frame with a balanced diet regime that consists of correct enough protein, carbohydrates, and wholesome fat. Proper nutrients helps muscle recovery and popular common standard performance.

eleven. Use Suitable Equipment:

When incorporating system which incorporates resistance bands or weights into your isometric training, pick out appropriate levels of resistance and make sure proper shape while the use of them.

12. Implement Proper Rest and Recovery:

Rest is critical for muscle repair and boom. Schedule rest days among excessive isometric physical games to permit your muscle organizations to get higher and adapt.

Important Considerations:

If you have have been given any pre-gift health conditions or accidents, discuss with a healthcare expert or a certified health teacher before beginning isometric training.

Focus on tremendous over quantity; perform isometric physical sports with manage and right approach instead of dashing via them.

Stop any workout right now if you enjoy sharp pain or pain.

By following these damage prevention suggestions and prioritizing your safety, you could experience the advantages of isometric schooling at the same time as minimizing the chance of accidents. Always pay attention on your body, do not forget of your limits, and make slow development to your workout workout routines. Remember that looking after your frame lets in you to hold pursuing your fitness goals in the end.

Chapter 9: Real-Life Success Stories

Testimonials from Isometric Training Enthusiasts

Isometric training has installation to be a transformative and empowering health approach for plenty people. Let's pay interest from some isometric schooling enthusiasts who have professional extremely good achievement of their fitness trips:

Testimonial 1 Sarah:

"After years of struggling to find out a exercise everyday that appropriate my busy time table, I stumbled upon isometric training. It has been a game-changer for me! The short but immoderate isometric bodily video video games healthy perfectly into my each day regular, allowing me to strengthen and tone my muscles with out spending hours on the fitness center. I've noticed big improvements in my center electricity and posture, and the super element is that I can do the ones bodily sports everywhere, whenever. Isometric schooling has made me revel in extra confident and empowered in my fitness journey!"

Testimonial 2 Mike:

"As a fitness fanatic, I become skeptical about isometric training on the start, thinking it may not be tough sufficient for my health degree. But as quickly as I blanketed isometric sports activities sports into my ordinary, I turn out to be blown away by using manner of the outcomes. The isometric holds not best stepped forward my electricity and muscle persistence, but furthermore they greater suitable my ordinary overall performance in unique kinds of education, like weightlifting and sports. Isometric schooling has taken my fitness to a whole new level, and I'm pleased with the profits I've made in my widespread athleticism."

Testimonial three Emily:

"As a person getting higher from a knee harm, I have end up searching out low-effect carrying events that could assist me rebuild strength without straining my joints. Isometric training come to be the fine solution. The static holds allowed me to paintings on my muscle power without

113

placing an excessive amount of pressure on my knees. Not most effective did I regain my power, but I additionally determined an improvement in my flexibility. Isometric training has given me hope and motivation to maintain my fitness adventure in spite of the traumatic situations I confronted."

Testimonial 4 David:

"As a hectic expert with restricted time for exercise, isometric schooling has been a lifesaver. The short and extreme sports have helped me hold my health even during the busiest days. I've been able to construct muscle and enhance my latest fitness degree with out spending hours on the fitness center. Isometric education has become an crucial a part of my each day regular, and I'm amazed at the effects I've finished on this type of brief time."

Testimonial 5 Jessica:

"Isometric training has surely converted my technique to health. As a yoga fanatic, I changed into intrigued thru the idea of isometric stretches. The static holds have not exceptional extended my flexibility but additionally provided a brand new length to my yoga exercise. I experience extra balanced, sturdy, and stage-headed in my poses. Isometric schooling has unlocked a deeper connection with my body, and I'm grateful for the newfound strength and mindfulness it has brought into my lifestyles."

Testimonial 6 Chris:

"Being a fitness beginner, I changed into intimidated thru traditional weightlifting and dynamic physical sports. Isometric schooling supplied a moderate yet powerful get right of entry to factor into the area of health. I started out with simple holds and frequently advanced to greater difficult variations. The self notion I received from my isometric exercise sports encouraged me to discover different styles of fitness. Now, I revel in more potent, greater lively, and endorsed to keep my health journey."

Chapter 10: Isometric Fundamentals

Stripping away needless gildings, we delve into the center factors of anatomy and body structure, dissecting the intricacies of muscle capabilities through the lens of simplicity; we discover the requirements that govern isometric training, emphasizing tangible information and smooth insights. This precursor lays the premise for a sensible exploration, imparting a whole understanding of the herbal underpinnings and guiding ideas that form the idea of an effective isometric education routine tailored for women.

The Basics of Anatomy and Physiology in Isometric Training

Understanding the mechanics of muscle mass and the way they reply to isometric training is essential for maximizing the benefits of your workout.

Let's begin with the basics. Muscles are the powerhouse of movement, permitting us to perform day by day sports and have interaction in diverse carrying activities.

Within the muscular gadget, sincerely one among kind varieties of muscles exists, together with skeletal muscle tissues, easy muscle organizations, and cardiac muscular tissues. For isometric carrying activities, our primary consciousness is on skeletal muscle businesses, the ones related to our bones that manage voluntary movements.

Now, allows delve a bit deeper into the shape of skeletal muscle tissue. Envision each muscle as a package deal of muscle fibers. These fibers contain smaller devices known as myofibrils, wherein the magic of muscle contraction happens. The fundamental unit of contraction is the sarcomere, a repeating unit alongside the myofibril chargeable for muscle shortening.

When you have got interaction in isometric physical games, you set off your muscle tissues without changing their period. In assessment to dynamic sporting sports activities that comprise motion, isometrics entail static contractions, wherein muscle groups generate pressure however do not visibly alternate in length. Grasping this concept is pivotal to knowledge the essence of isometric training.

Moving at once to the body shape of muscle contraction, it's far important to acquaint yourself with the neuromuscular junction. This is in which nerves talk with muscle tissues. When you make a decision to flex a muscle sooner or later of an isometric exercising, your thoughts send indicators thru your nerves, triggering the release of neurotransmitters that stimulate muscle contraction.

Now, allows discover the function of blood go together with the waft and oxygen shipping in the course of isometric sports activities. As muscle tissue settlement, they in brief compress blood vessels, reducing blood go with the flow and inflicting a buildup of metabolic byproducts like lactic acid. This herbal machine contributes to the general effectiveness of isometric physical video games.

Understanding the energy systems at play is also vital. Isometric sports activities mainly faucet into the anaerobic energy machine, which can no longer depend on oxygen. This system provides brief bursts of energy, making isometrics an inexperienced preference for quick, immoderate sporting sports.

By acknowledging how muscle mass characteristic at a crucial degree, individuals can higher harness the benefits of isometric education. Get organized to interact your muscle corporations intelligently and make the maximum of your exercise routine with the aid of the usage of facts the problematic dance amongst anatomy and body form.

Exploring the Principles of Isometric Training

Having protected the foundational factors of anatomy and frame shape, it's now time to delve into the necessities that make isometric education a dynamic and effective method to improving strength and standard fitness.

Principle 1: Time below Tension

Isometric bodily sports revolve spherical keeping a muscle contraction for an extended duration, a idea known as time below anxiety (TUT). Unlike dynamic physical sports in which muscle tissue agreement and make bigger, isometrics focus on a sustained contraction, intensifying the engagement of muscle fibers. This prolonged tension triggers metabolic responses, promoting muscle growth and staying strength.

Principle 2: Progressive Overload

To witness non-stop improvement, it is vital to steadily undertaking your muscle businesses. Progressive overload in isometric education includes step by step growing the depth or length of your contractions this need to suggest which include resistance in case you're the usage of props, or preserving the contraction for an extended duration. By step by step overloading your muscle groups, you stimulate non-forestall model, fostering power income over the years.

Principle 3: Specificity of Training

Isometric wearing activities offer the opportunity to intention particular muscular tissues or muscle organizations with precision. Whether you're aiming to tone your hands, toughen your middle, or beautify your leg muscle companies, specificity in education guarantees you awareness at the regions you want to enhance. This targeted approach makes isometrics flexible, allowing you to tailor your recurring to satisfy your particular fitness desires.

Principle four: Mind-Muscle Connection

Connecting your mind collectively with your muscle organizations is a important trouble of isometric schooling. By concentrating on the muscle you're attractive and preserving highbrow popularity in some unspecified time within the future of the contraction, you decorate the effectiveness of the workout. This thoughts-muscle connection now not first-rate improves the excellent of your exercising however moreover promotes better normal body attention.

Principle five: Rest and Recovery

Just like another form of exercising, true enough rest and recovery are crucial for pinnacle-rated consequences. Isometric schooling induces micro-tears in muscle fibers, and they want time to restore and develop more potent. Be privy to your body's alerts, make certain right sleep, and incorporate relaxation days into your recurring to allow your muscle corporations to get better sincerely.

Principle 6: Breathing Techniques

Proper respiration is regularly not noted but plays a essential function in isometric bodily video games. Maintain a controlled and consistent respiration sample at some stage in contractions to make sure regular oxygen deliver in your muscle groups. Deep breaths can also help you keep attention and decrease useless anxiety, permitting you to get the maximum out of every isometric maintain.

Principle 7: Safety First

Lastly, commonly prioritize safety. Whether you're a newbie or an experienced health enthusiast, right form is paramount. Ensure you're in a strong position, especially if appearing status or weight-bearing isometrics. Listen in your frame, keep away from overexertion, and talk with a health professional if you have any concerns about your shape or suitability for specific wearing occasions.

These ideas from the bedrock of effective isometric schooling for women By incorporating those into your recurring, you may no longer most effective supply a boost to your muscle corporations however additionally empower yourself with a bendy and attractive method to health. Embrace those standards, live regular, and enjoy the transformative advantages of isometric sports activities for your adventure to a more potent and extra wholesome you!

Chapter 11: Preparing For Isometric Workouts

Before we leap into the sensible stuff, allows lay the foundation. Checking how fit your needs are permits make your exercising stable and effective. Also, installing an high-quality exercise vicinity makes sticking to this healthful exercise a good deal much less complicated. This chapter offers easy guidelines and steps to guide you via the start, offering a sturdy base on your isometric sports activities. Now, permits talk approximately the practical topics, understand your competencies, and set up an wonderful place in your properly-being.

Checking Fitness Levels

Starting isometric physical sports activities is exciting, and the first step is to peer how fit you are. These permits make a exercising plan that suits your strengths and areas to enhance.

Think about your common fitness. Are there any health problems you want to be careful about? Isometric sports activities are generally solid, however it is well to reflect on consideration on any fitness troubles you've got got. If you aren't certain, speak me to a healthcare professional is a brilliant concept.

Now, allow's smash down the fitness check:

Cardio Health:

A sturdy coronary heart is crucial for normal fitness. Think about sports that make your heart beat quicker. Can you climb stairs without feeling tired? Try a brisk stroll or light jog for 10-15 minutes and study how your frame reacts. This lets in set a place to begin in your coronary heart fitness.

Strength and Muscle Endurance:

Strength is important for isometric wearing activities. Test your muscular tissues with fundamental sporting activities like push-americaor squats. How lengthy are you able to preserve a plank? These easy exams display what your muscle corporations can do and help you begin at the right stage.

Flexibility:

Flexibility is regularly forgotten however topics lots. Try conducting on your toes or doing clean yoga poses. Checking flexibility allows locate regions that need attention and prevents accidents in awesome sports activities.

Balance and Coordination:

Isometric bodily sports want stability, so take a look at your balance. Stand on one leg for 30 seconds and word if you wobble. Try clean coordination wearing sports like marching in place. These checks supply an first rate concept of your bodily skills.

Joint Health:

Think about your joints—they may be essential for movement. Notice any ache or stiffness in advantageous areas. It's important to select wearing sports nice to your joints and adjust your normal if wanted.

This check isn't always approximately evaluating or judging but is a beneficial guide to your fitness journey. With this records, you can plan isometric sporting occasions that healthful your capabilities and gradually enhance as you get more potent. If any problems arise, speaking to a healthcare professional guarantees a constant and fun health revel in. Now which you've checked your health, allow's flow directly to developing a regular exercising area in phase three.2. Ready for the following step?

Building a Safe Workout Space

Now that you comprehend your health ranges and are organized for isometric wearing activities, the following vital step is to create a secure exercising vicinity. Having an environment that permits you hobby, stay stable, and be regular is prime to a a success isometric exercise normal.

Here's a guide to help set up the precise exercise area:

1. Choose a Dedicated Area:

Pick a particular spot in your private home for isometric workout workouts. It may want to now not want to be massive, but having a dedicated vicinity makes it clear that it's time to exercise. Make high-quality it is nicely-ventilated and free from distractions.

2. Clear the Clutter:

Keep your exercise location freed from boundaries. Remove anything that would experience you up. A easy and prepared place no longer handiest makes it extra secure however also helps you to pass with out issues sooner or later of sports.

3. Invest in Proper Flooring:

Think approximately the floors in your exercising vicinity. If possible, pick out a ground that offers a piece at the same time as you step on it. Exercise mats or foam floors are top notch for defensive your joints at some stage in isometric sports activities.

4. Good Lighting:

Having sufficient moderate is essential for safety and attention. Natural moderate is high-quality, however if this isn't viable, get colourful, strength-green lighting to your exercise vicinity. This no longer excellent helps you note higher but additionally boosts your temper and motivation.

5. Ventilation:

Make positive there is exquisite airflow on your workout region. Proper air waft maintains you from getting too hot and enables you live snug in some unspecified time in the destiny of sporting sports activities. If you're inside, open home windows or use a fan to hold a nice temperature.

6. Mirror, Mirror on the Wall:

Having a reflect for your workout space can be useful. It lets you take a look at your shape and posture, ensuring you are doing each isometric workout proper. This visual comments makes your workout extra powerful.

7. Gather Your Equipment:

Depending on the isometric sports activities you are doing, get any wished tool earlier of time. Whether it's miles resistance bands, dumbbells, or balance balls, having the whole lot prepared saves time and maintains your ordinary ordinary.

eight. Create a Positive Atmosphere:

Make your exercise region personal. Add topics that encourage and encourage you, like upbeat tune, costs, or your preferred exercise equipment. A exceptional environment makes isometric wearing sports activities extra thrilling.

nine. Establish a Routine:

Being everyday is critical for any fitness journey. Set particular times on your isometric exercise workouts and stay with it slow desk. This now not nice allows make it a addiction but additionally makes high first-rate you placed aside time on your health.

By growing a space that suits you, you are making an environment wherein isometric sporting activities can artwork properly. This cautious method makes positive you are consistent, no longer distracted, and in a high-quality mind-set in the course of your sporting events. Now that your workout region is ready, you are ready to start your isometric workout ordinary with self belief. Excited to start your exercising exercises in this properly-organized vicinity?

Chapter 12: Unveiling The Power Of Isometric Exercises

Unlocking a stronger, greater toned frame would possibly now not always call for constant motion; in fact, the name of the sport also can lie inside the strength of stillness. This chapter explores the captivating worldwide of isometric sports sports particularly designed for women. Forget the misconception that fitness necessitates perpetual movement. Here, we gift an intensive manual to sculpting robust shoulders, properly-defined palms, effective legs, and business enterprise glutes—during the artwork of maintaining every day. No want for tough sporting activities; surely the simplicity of isometrics to spark transformative modifications in your frame. Get geared up to encompass a fitness method that demonstrates energy inside the stillness of controlled contractions. Let's dive into the information!

Isometrics for the Upper Body

Let's delve into the crucial elements of upper frame isometrics and apprehend how they may be able to benefit you.

Building Strong Shoulders and Toned Arms

Shoulder Stability:

Begin work for your pinnacle frame through specializing in constructing sturdy and strong shoulders. Isometric physical activities interact your shoulder muscle groups with out the need for repetitive actions, making them first-class for joint-nice exercising sporting events. An tremendous exercise to acquire that is the isometric shoulder press.

Start with the useful resource of popularity collectively together with your ft shoulder-width apart, retaining a weight or resistance band at shoulder peak. Push upwards in competition to the resistance, attractive your shoulder muscle tissues, and hold for a depend of 10-15 seconds. This not handiest targets your deltoids but additionally complements commonplace shoulder balance.

Toning Arms:

Moving on to the arms, isometric bicep and tricep sports activities activities are extraordinary for sculpting and firming with out excessive bulk. Try the isometric bicep curl by the use of the use of retaining a dumbbell in each hand, palms going via in advance. Keep your elbows near your frame, curl the weights midway up, and preserve the place. This concentrates anxiety for your biceps, promoting muscle definition.

For triceps, the isometric tricep kickback is your bypass-to. Stand with a dumbbell in your proper hand, hinge ahead on the hips, and increase your arm again. Hold this function, feeling the burn on your triceps, and repeat on the alternative aspect. These wearing activities, with their static holds, correctly activate your muscle mass for a extra toned and smooth look.

Sculpting Defined Back Muscles

A sturdy, defined back not best improves your posture but additionally contributes to an wellknown sculpted look. Isometric physical video games offer an excellent manner of engaging in this, specifically with the isometric pull-up.

Using a strong horizontal bar, feature your hands shoulder-width apart with fingers dealing with faraway from you. Jump up, then slowly decrease yourself halfway down and preserve for so long as you could. This dreams your latissimus dorsi and rhomboid muscle tissues, fostering a nicely-described and toned over again.

Additionally, the isometric row is extremely good for focused on your center and pinnacle lower again muscles. Using resistance bands or weights, hinge at your hips and pull the resistance towards your chest, protecting for several seconds. This no longer simplest improves your again muscle tissues but additionally engages your center for added benefits.

Incorporating these better body isometric wearing activities into your recurring will now not simplest toughen and tone your shoulders and palms but moreover make contributions to an normal balanced frame. Consistency is prime, so make the ones carrying occasions a everyday part of your health routine for lasting and good sized results.

Isometrics for the Lower Body

Let's now test out numerous isometric carrying sports that specialize in building powerful legs and sculpting organization glutes. Get equipped to experience the burn in all the right locations as you embark in this journey to beautify and tone your lower body.

Building Powerful Legs

Quadriceps Dominance:

Let's kick topics off through using highlighting the robust quadriceps, the muscle mass on the the front of your thighs. Isometric sporting sports activities can efficaciously intention those muscle businesses, selling power and definition. The isometric wall sit is a traditional example that calls for no system.

Find a strong wall and reduce yourself proper right into a seated function, together with your knees forming a 90-degree mind-set. Hold this characteristic for so long as you may, feeling the burn for your quadriceps. This exercising no longer super strengthens your quads however moreover engages your middle and glutes.

Hamstring Engagement:

For a well-rounded lower frame exercising, it is crucial to interact your hamstrings. Isometric hamstring curls may be completed the use of a stability ball. Lie to your again collectively together with your heels on the ball, enhance your hips, and roll the ball in the direction of you the usage of your feet. Hold the virtually shriveled position, attractive your hamstrings, after which roll the ball decrease lower back out. This exercising desires your hamstrings and glutes, fostering balance in your decrease frame muscle improvement.

Calf Definition:

Completing the trio of leg muscle tissue, the calves deserve interest too. Isometric calf will increase are an effective way to construct definition for your calf muscle tissues. Stand on the threshold of a step, enhance your heels, and hold the vicinity for 10-15 seconds. This exercise now not only goals your calf muscle companies however moreover complements ankle stability.

Sculpting Firm Glutes

Glute Activation:

Now, allow's shift our reputation to sculpting the ones organisation glutes that beautify your everyday silhouette. Isometric glute bridges are a superb way to prompt and enhance your glute muscle corporations. Lie for your lower back collectively together with your knees bent, increase your hips towards the ceiling, and maintain the location. Squeeze your glutes at the top and feel the burn in your posterior chain. This workout no longer only tones your glutes but moreover improves hip stability.

Lunges with a Twist:

Isometric lunges take the conventional lunge up a notch. Step beforehand right right into a lunge function, however rather than transferring up and down, hold the lunge role for an prolonged duration. This engages your glutes and quadriceps, presenting a difficult but effective workout in your lower frame.

Inner and Outer Thighs:

To entire your lower frame sculpting, don't forget isometric adductor and abductor carrying sports. Using a resistance band, carry out side leg will increase on the identical time as reputation to purpose your abductors. For adductors, sit down at the ground together along with your legs prolonged and vicinity the band spherical your ankles, then push your legs outward against the resistance. These sporting sports make contributions to the sculpting of your internal and outer thighs, promoting a balanced lower frame look.

Incorporating those decrease body isometric sports into your recurring will now not fantastic build strength and definition in your legs and glutes but additionally enhance ordinary lower body balance. Remember to take note of your body, start at a snug stage, and regularly increase depth as you improvement for your fitness journey.

Chapter 13: Personalizing Your Isometric Workout

Did that isometric wearing sports may be the critical detail to achieving your health desires? In this financial wreck, we're going to discover the power of customization and smooth integration. Whether you're aiming for power, flexibility, or really want to function a few spices in your ordinary, isometrics offer a bendy solution. Customize your exercise to healthy your goals with the aid of using blending static holds into your present fitness routine. Get ready to look how this easy yet powerful approach can decorate your fitness experience. Are you equipped to unharness the capacity of isometric physical video games and reshape your exercise plan?

Tailoring Workouts to Meet Your Goals

Isometric sports, with their but contractions and mild impact, are an awesome choice for ladies looking for to adapt their fitness bodily sports to particular desires. In this phase, we're going to explore the ability of isometric sports and the way adjusting them to person desires can enhance your regular fitness adventure.

Understanding Your Goals:

Before beginning your isometric everyday, it's far essential to apprehend your fitness dreams, whether or now not it is building strength, improving posture, or handling pressure. Isometric sports activities sports cater to severa desires, and via defining yours, you placed the extent for a custom designed and effective exercise plan.

Building Strength and Tone:

If your essential intention is to construct strength and tone your muscle mass, isometric bodily sports activities offer a very particular technique. These physical video video games contain preserving a static characteristic, growing anxiety in unique muscle businesses. For instance, wall sits, planks, or static lunges may be protected to engage most vital muscle groups, selling strength improvement and definition.

When customizing your ordinary, recollect the duration of every isometric preserve. For those focusing on electricity, shorter, greater immoderate holds may be beneficial. It's approximately finding the proper balance to assignment your muscle mass without compromising shape.

Improving Endurance:

Isometric sporting activities additionally may be tailor-made to beautify staying energy. By extending the duration of every keep and incorporating loads of positions, you could decorate your muscle tissues' stamina. Gradually growing preserve times and such as a combination of carrying events like static squats, plank variations, and isometric push-u.S.A.Will make a contribution to advanced staying strength over the years.

Enhancing Flexibility:

Flexibility is a few other trouble that may be addressed thru isometric physical video games. While no longer as dynamic as some flexibility-focused sporting activities, isometrics can assist improve joint form of motion and ordinary flexibility. Incorporating positions that emphasize stretching and elongating muscle mass, which encompass isometric lunges or hamstring stretches, can contribute to stepped forward flexibility through the years.

Targeting Specific Areas:

One of the good sized blessings of isometric physical video games is their capacity to aim unique muscle agencies. Tailor your ordinary to attention on areas which can be especially vital to you. For instance, if you want to strengthen your center, embody isometric bodily sports just like the plank or the boat pose. If you're in search of to tone your arms, consist of static holds like wall push-americaor bicep curls.

Customizing Intensity:

Another manner to tailor isometric exercising routines is thru adjusting the intensity. Beginners might also moreover start with shorter holds and much less repetitions, regularly growing as they emerge as extra comfortable. Advanced practitioners can mission themselves with longer holds and further complicated positions, making sure endured development aligned with their health desires.

Listen to Your Body:

While customization is essential, it's miles in addition critical to concentrate on your body. If an workout reasons pain beyond the everyday burn associated with isometrics, alter for that reason or visit a health professional. Every female's frame is particular, and the essential component to a a hit isometric routine lies in finding the stableness amongst mission and luxury.

Tailoring isometric exercise exercises to man or woman dreams entails records what you need to obtain, choosing appropriate physical video games, and customizing intensity and period. By incorporating the ones customized elements, you could make isometric sports activities a powerful and exciting a part of your fitness journey.

Incorporating Isometrics into Your Current Fitness Routine:

Now that we've were given explored tailoring isometric wearing activities to person desires, allow's take a look at seamlessly integrating the ones powerful static contractions into your present day-day fitness everyday. Whether you are a normal health club-goer, a yoga enthusiast, or a person with an established recurring, together with isometrics can bring a latest dimension in your health journey.

Isometrics as Additional Exercises:

Isometric physical video video games can feature exceptional additions for your cutting-edge exercise normal. For aerobic enthusiasts, incorporating isometrics should make more potent muscle corporations without immoderate effect on joints, this is specifically useful for immoderate-impact sports like running or aerobics.

For the ones already engaged in energy education, isometrics provide a completely precise form of muscle engagement. By introducing static holds or isometric versions of traditional bodily video games, collectively with static lunges or isometric squats, you can goal muscle agencies in a remarkable way, promoting regular strength and stability.

Integrating Isometrics into Yoga Practices:

Yoga practitioners can also benefit from which consist of isometric sports activities. While yoga certainly consists of diverse static poses, consisting of unique isometric holds can intensify the exercise. Including isometric versions of conventional poses, like a static warrior pose or plank versions, can enhance the electricity and stability additives of your yoga ordinary.

Moreover, isometrics can enhance the mind-body connection that yoga emphasizes. Focusing on muscle engagement and breath manage during isometric holds aligns well with the thoughts of mindfulness and attention in yoga.

Blending Isometrics with Pilates:

For dedicated Pilates enthusiasts, integrating isometric carrying sports activities seamlessly complements the center-strengthening consciousness of this situation. Adding static holds, which include an isometric bridge or plank, enhances center engagement, contributing to advanced stability and stability. The managed and unique movements inherent in Pilates align nicely with the deliberate nature of isometric wearing activities.

Creating Isometric Circuits:

Another powerful manner to comprise isometrics into your present regular is with the aid of using way of developing committed isometric circuits. Designing a circuit that combines traditional wearing sports with isometric holds can offer a entire exercising. For example, pair dynamic moves like squats or lunges with static holds like wall sits or plank variations.

This approach now not handiest continues your ordinary dynamic and attractive but moreover ensures a properly-rounded exercise that addresses each dynamic and static muscle engagement.

Balancing Isometric and Dynamic Exercises:

Balance is fundamental whilst incorporating isometrics into your modern-day health ordinary. While isometrics offer particular blessings, they should now not update dynamic actions really. Striking a stability amongst dynamic sporting sports and isometric holds ensures that you aim muscular tissues in severa techniques, selling not unusual strength, flexibility, and staying power.

Progressive Integration:

If you're new to isometric physical games, keep in mind progressively integrating them into your normal. Start with a few isometric holds in line with session and often increase the length and intensity as your frame adapts. This gradual incorporation permits your muscle organizations and joints to acclimate to the static contractions, decreasing the threat of overexertion.

Incorporating isometrics into your existing health everyday offers a myriad of blessings, from better muscle engagement to diverse exercise physical games. Whether you are a seasoned health enthusiast or just starting your adventure, isometric carrying sports can seamlessly turn out to be a precious trouble of your commonplace health habitual.

Chapter 14: The Strength Of Still Yoga

Did that combining easy however effective isometric wearing occasions with yoga can change your health enjoy? Get ready for a massive revelation in our next economic disaster - a clean combination we name Still Yoga. Step into an area where muscle companies artwork with precision, conventional yoga poses get stronger, and quick workout routines go away an enduring affect. Imagine gaining power, flexibility, and mindfulness suddenly. The secret is within the interesting mixture searching in advance to you inside the next pages. Brace your self to locate The Strength of Still Yoga and see your health ordinary change.

Blending Isometrics with Yoga Poses

Still Yoga is a strong aggregate of traditional isometric physical sports and historical yoga, creating an entire way to live bodily nicely. In this segment, we'll discover the benefits that display up while isometrics integrate with yoga poses, giving start to what we lovingly name "The Strength of Still Yoga."

Isometric physical sports activities mean squeezing precise muscle groups without changing their length or joint attitude, presenting a very particular type of resistance. This idea smoothly fits with the idea of yoga, which is about stability, flexibility, and mindfulness. Combining the ones two practices outcomes in a workout that includes every the frame and mind.

As you start your Still Yoga adventure, you'll discover that traditional yoga poses may be advanced by way of the usage of including isometric squeezes. For example, inside the direction of a traditional yoga pose like Warrior II, squeezing your muscle groups on the same time as retaining the pose ought to make it extra intense, activating muscle businesses extra efficiently.

The Strength of Still Yoga comes from its functionality to purpose specific muscle tissue with precision. By adding isometric squeezes to yoga poses, you now not simplest make the exercise extra severe but additionally art work your muscular tissues in a way that conventional yoga by myself may not. This targeted attempt can result in better muscle tone and power, assisting you form your frame.

Moreover, mixing isometrics with yoga improves stability and stability. Isometric squeezes make you prompt and aid stabilizing muscular tissues, becoming properly with yoga's cognizance on balance. This combined method allows you understand and manipulate your body higher.

One of the advantages of The Strength of Still Yoga is how green it's far with time. Busy schedules frequently make it difficult to exercise regularly, however Still Yoga gives an answer. The depth of isometric squeezes allows for shorter however effective exercising sporting events. This way you could get the advantages of isometrics and yoga in a short time, making it easy to in form into your each day recurring.

As you find out the location of Still Yoga, you can phrase a more potent connection amongst your thoughts and frame. The mindfulness from conventional yoga is boosted with the useful resource of using the focus favored at some point of isometric squeezes. This syncing of breath, motion, and muscle engagement now not handiest will increase physical benefits but additionally reduces stress and promotes highbrow readability.

The Strength of Still Yoga goes beyond normal exercising sporting activities. It introduces a dynamic combination of isometric squeezes into the calm flow of yoga, ensuing in a exercising that no longer only improves power and flexibility however moreover nurtures mindfulness and balance. As you encompass this aggregate, you could discover yourself on a journey to a more healthy, greater balanced you.

6.2 Boosting Flexibility and Strength Together

Welcome to Still Yoga, where the fusion of power and versatility takes the spotlight. In this section, we discover the exceptional teamwork that takes place while you beautify each factors on the identical time, providing a whole method to staying bodily nicely.

Flexibility and electricity are regularly visible as opposites, however Still Yoga breaks down those obstacles, displaying they will paintings together. Traditional yoga is known for enhancing flexibility with dynamic stretches and poses. On the opportunity hand, isometric sporting sports consciousness on building electricity by using enticing muscle tissues with out movement. The magic takes vicinity whilst those two practices come together.

Isometric squeezes in yoga poses create a completely unique venture on your muscle companies. Take the Forward Fold, for instance. By together with isometric squeezes, like urgent your palms collectively or appealing your middle at the same time as retaining the pose, you no longer most effective stretch more but additionally spark off and improve the muscle tissues. This dual movement boosts every flexibility and strength, growing a greater balanced and sturdy frame.

The key to this double development is in proprioceptive neuromuscular facilitation (PNF). Still Yoga makes use of PNF thoughts via appealing a muscle organization and then stretching it extra at a few degree within the relaxation section. This verbal exchange improves flexibility and strengthens the muscle groups of their newly stretched kingdom. The quit give up result is a dynamic interplay that blessings your body as a whole.

As you upload isometrics in your yoga habitual, you'll have a observe a huge impact on joint balance. Isometric squeezes make you spark off stabilizing muscle mass spherical joints, improving joint balance. This balance not handiest will growth your traditional sort of movement but additionally lowers the hazard of injuries, making your health revel in greater solid and extra powerful.

Still Yoga's technique to boosting flexibility and power is going past physical benefits. The targeted engagement needed for the duration of isometric squeezes creates a deeper connection amongst your thoughts and body. As you go with the flow thru poses with intentional muscle engagement, your recognition of your frame's abilties and barriers grows, number one to higher body manipulate.

Another amazing element of enhancing flexibility and strength collectively is the overall overall performance it brings to your exercises. Regular sporting activities often separate flexibility and strength education education, worrying more time. Still Yoga simplifies this, offering a whole exercising in a shorter time. This efficient approach makes it less tough to in shape into busy schedules even as getting maximum outcomes.

The fusion of flexibleness and strength in Still Yoga gives a whole approach to health. By combining the dynamic stretches of yoga with the static intensity of isometric squeezes, you not simplest beautify your bodily abilties however furthermore nurture a deeper thoughts-body connection. Step into the arena where flexibility and strength come together, and word the transformative energy of Still Yoga in every stretch and squeeze.

Chapter 15: 10-Minute Quick Workouts For Busy Women

Did you understand that such as quick bursts of although sporting sports to your busy day can convey first rate health benefits? In this bankruptcy, we discover the power of fast, targeted however sports for ladies at the glide. Fact: Still bodily games paintings many muscle groups even as now not having lengthy classes. Can certainly 10 mins change your fitness routine? Get equipped to discover clean routines made to your lifestyles, presenting a sensible way to construct power, tone up, and improve strength. What if unlocking your body's skills changed into much less complicated than you idea? Let's explore the transformative effect of time-saving even though wearing events.

10-Minute Quick Workouts

Life can be busy, and locating time for a protracted exercising ordinary can be tough. However, with those short however physical sports, you may make massive improvement within the course of your health dreams in only a bit of your day.

Still physical games endorse contracting muscle mass with out shifting the joints, best for immediate and effective exercise physical games. The 10-minute period of these workouts fits with out difficulty into your busy time table, so you can awareness on your health with out dropping precious time.

Understanding Still Exercises

Before stepping into the correct workout exercises, let's quick recognize nevertheless sporting sports. Unlike everyday physical games with repeated movements, although sports activities attention on maintaining a feature, selling energy and staying power.

The actual issue approximately but bodily sports is their flexibility. Whether you are at domestic, at art work, or journeying, you can do those bodily video games with out precise system. This makes them an tremendous preference for busy girls with out get entry to to a gymnasium or prolonged time for a exercising.

The 10-Minute Still Routine

1. Warm-up (1 minute): Start with light cardio, like marching in region or moderate leaping jacks, to boom blood float and prepare your muscles for the upcoming though sporting sports.

2. Wall Sit (2 minutes): Find a sturdy wall and slide down until your knees are bent at a ninety-diploma attitude. Hold this position, working your quadriceps and glutes. This exercise is terrific for toning your lower frame and constructing endurance.

three. Plank (2 minutes): Move to a plank function, supporting your body to your ft and forearms. Engage your center muscle tissues, preserving your frame in a proper away line. Planks are exceptional for strengthening your center and enhancing normal balance.

4. Chair Squats (2 mins): Use a strong chair for managed squats, decreasing your body as

despite the fact that sitting down. Focus on going for walks your leg muscle agencies in the course of the movement. Chair squats target your quads, hamstrings, and glutes.

five. Still Bicep Curl (2 mins): Grab a couple of mild dumbbells or family objects. Hold them at shoulder top, elbows bent at a ninety-diploma attitude. Keep this characteristic, attractive your biceps. This workout dreams your arm muscle groups with out complex actions.

Cool Down (1 minute): Finish the everyday with moderate stretching to decorate flexibility and help muscle recuperation.

These 10-minute although exercise exercises provide a brief but effective solution for busy girls looking for to feature fitness to their every day lives. Focus on suitable form and controlled movements for the first rate effects. Stay regular, and you could quickly see the tremendous effect of those brief however powerful classes to your usual properly-being.

Still Exercises for Office Breaks

Now, permit's discover even though wearing sports designed for quick office breaks. It's time to reveal the ones sitting moments into opportunities to refresh your frame and thoughts.

The Sitting Challenge

In modern fast artwork environment, it's miles commonplace to discover yourself sitting for a long term. Office jobs that comprise sitting masses can have an effect for your health, causing issues like terrible posture and muscle stiffness. However, with some strategic nevertheless sports activities, you could counteract the horrible consequences of sitting too lengthy and upload bursts of energy to your workday.

Benefits of Still Exercises in the course of Office Breaks

Before we get into specific carrying sports, let's see why even though physical sports are great in your workplace ordinary. Isometrics will permit you to art work many muscle companies and now not the use of a need lots area or unique gadget. You can discreetly upload those physical games in your breaks, promoting circulate, decreasing muscle anxiety, and boosting everyday electricity ranges.

Office Break Still Routine

1. Desk Push-ups (2 minutes): Stand some steps some distance from your table, location your fingers shoulder-width apart on the edge, and lean in. Lower your chest towards the table and keep off up. This push-up version targets your chest, shoulders, and triceps.

2. Seated Leg Raise (2 mins): While sitting at your desk, straighten one or both legs and maintain in area for a few seconds. Lower the leg(s) backpedal with out letting them contact the ground. This exercise engages your center and works your lower belly muscle tissues.

3. Cubicle Wall Sit (2 mins): Find an empty area in competition to a cubicle wall and slide down right into a sitting function together with your knees at a ninety-degree attitude. This despite the fact that squat engages your quadriceps and glutes, countering the consequences of sitting too long.

4. Chair Dips (2 minutes): Using the brink of your place of job chair, function your arms on each detail of your hips. Slide your backside off the chair and lower your frame, then maintain off up. Chair dips intention your triceps and are excellent for toning your hands.

five. Still Neck Stretch (2 minutes): Gently tilt your head to at least one factor, bringing your ear towards your shoulder, and maintain the stretch for 30 seconds. Repeat on the alternative aspect. This exercising lets in relieve tension within the neck and shoulders.

Adding Still Exercises to Your Workday

Consistency is crucial to get the advantages of these administrative center destroy even though sports activities. Try to characteristic them in your each day habitual, perhaps inside the direction of brief breaks or possibly at some stage in virtual conferences wherein you can quietly do these moves. By doing this, you will not best decorate your physical nicely-being but additionally beautifies intellectual clarity and productiveness all through your workday.

Chapter 16: Eating Right And Isometric Exercise

Did you recognize that to get the most from your isometric exercises, it is now not pretty a wonderful deal the way you flow into however moreover about what you consume and the way you cope with your body? In this financial disaster, we're going to find out the era inside the returned of ways nutrients, staying hydrated, and recuperation techniques can beautify the effectiveness of isometric education, specifically for girls. From the importance of getting a extraordinary mix of proteins, carbs, and fat to retaining your muscle tissues hydrated, we're capable of percentage practical suggestions to make your isometric bodily games even higher. Get ready to test the crucial basics that will help you fuel your frame effectively and enhance your consequences in isometric bodily games.

Providing the Right Fuel for Isometric Success

Success in isometric sporting activities isn't always just about the physical effort; it's also about giving your frame the right gas for better overall performance and outcomes. In this detail, we will talk the crucial hyperlink between what you consume and isometric schooling, guiding you on a manner to gasoline your body for fulfillment on your isometric sports activities.

Understanding the Connection amongst Nutrition and Isometric Training

Isometric carrying sports want a special blend of muscle power and persistence. While doing those static contractions, your muscle agencies want a non-stop energy deliver to carry out properly. Good nutrients is important to offer this electricity and help your muscle tissues during isometric physical video video games.

Balanced Nutrients

Make tremendous your weight loss plan consists of a aggregate of proteins, carbs, and fat. Proteins help in muscle repair and growth, carbs supply the electricity wished for isometric contractions, and healthy fats contribute to normal body features.

Protein for Muscle Health

Proteins are crucial for anyone doing isometric sporting sports because of the reality they construct and repair muscle mass. Include lean protein assets like chook, fish, tofu, and legumes to your weight-reduction plan. These food help your muscle corporations get better after hard isometric intervals.

Using Carbs as Energy

Carbs are the primary strength deliver to your frame, specially in some unspecified time within the destiny of severe sports activities like isometric wearing events. Choose complicated carbs like entire grains, culmination, and vegetables for a constant launch of energy, supporting you maintain your exercise. This sustained electricity is important for holding isometric contractions over a long length.

Staying Hydrated and Electrolytes

Keeping hydrated is critical for maximum ordinary performance in isometric bodily sports. Water is important for commonplace health and lets in hold muscle characteristic and joint flexibility. Also, bear in mind replenishing out of area electrolytes, specifically within the route of intense isometric workout routines. Drinks with electrolytes or herbal property like coconut water can assist repair the stableness.

Meal Timing and Isometric Workouts

When you consume can notably impact your isometric schooling. Having a balanced meal a few hours in advance than your consultation ensures your frame has the nutrients it goals. Also, a placed up-exercise meal with protein and carbs allows with muscle healing and restores energy.

Pre-Workout Eating

Eat a moderate meal with every carbs and proteins approximately 2-three hours in advance than your isometric exercising. This gives a everyday launch of electricity for the duration of your consultation, stopping fatigue.

Post-Workout Eating

After your isometric ordinary, reason for a post-exercise meal or snack within the first hour. This have to consist of each proteins and carbs to kickstart muscle restoration and top off glycogen stores.

To sum up, the connection amongst vitamins and isometric training is crucial. Choosing the proper nutrients at the right time now not quality boosts your general overall performance all through isometric sporting events but moreover enables muscle recovery and ordinary nicely-being. Make considerate selections to your healthy eating plan, stay hydrated, and witness your isometric success as your body receives the only fuel it desires.

Staying Hydrated and Recovering Well

Hydration and recovery play vital roles in a a fulfillment isometric training plan. Ensuring your frame gets enough fluids and the use of effective restoration strategies could make a large difference on your ordinary usual overall performance and nicely-being. Let's discover why hydration and healing rely inside the context of isometric physical activities.

Hydration Essentials for Isometric Success

Understanding Fluid Balance

Hydration isn't always pretty lots quenching your thirst; it's far approximately preserving the right balance of fluids to your body. This balance is critical for isometric sports. When you do static contractions, your muscle groups generate heat, and right hydration permits use up this warm temperature, stopping overheating and selling most wonderful muscle characteristic.

Water because the Foundation

Water is the number one detail for hydration, and its significance can not be overstated. It lubricates joints, transports nutrients to cells, and allows regulate body temperature – all important for a achievement isometric training. Aim to drink water constantly sooner or later of the day, now not just eventually of your workout.

Individual Hydration Needs

The amount of water you need can range based mostly on factors like body weight, weather, and the intensity of your isometric ordinary. A contemporary guideline is to eat at the least 8 eight-ounce glasses of water a day, however character dreams can also additionally differ. Listen to your body – in case you sense thirsty, drink, and be aware about your urine coloration, aiming for a diminished yellow color.

Effective Hydration Strategies at some stage in Isometric Workouts

Sip, Don't Guzzle

Rather than ingesting some of water right away, sip it all through your isometric exercising. This prevents overloading your belly and minimizes the risk of pain. Small, everyday sips ensure a regular consumption, maintaining you thoroughly hydrated without inflicting digestive issues at some point of your bodily video games.

Balancing Electrolytes

In addition to water, be aware of your electrolyte balance, particularly in case you sweat loads in the course of isometric sports activities. Electrolytes like sodium, potassium, and magnesium are important for muscle contraction and fluid balance. Consider which consist of electrolyte-rich drinks or snacks, particularly in case your exercising exercises are prolonged or excessive.

Post-Workout Hydration

Rehydrating after your isometric session is similarly critical. Your frame loses fluids through sweat within the direction of workout, and replenishing the ones out of location fluids is essential for healing. Aim to devour water or a hydrating beverage inside the first hour after your exercising to useful aid the recuperation device.

Prioritizing Recovery for Optimal Isometric Results

Understanding the Importance of Recovery

Isometric sporting sports placed a whole lot of pressure for your muscle agencies, and prioritizing healing is prime to preventing fatigue, minimizing soreness, and getting the maximum from your sports. Incorporate powerful restoration techniques into your recurring to make certain your muscle groups are organized for the subsequent isometric project.

Chapter 17: Unveiling The Relationship Between Mind

Did you ever keep in mind that the important thing to cultivating a greater in shape thoughts might likely lie in the depth of your muscle contractions? In this ninth installment of our exploration into Isometric Exercises for Women, we are able to resolve the complicated connection a number of the thoughts and frame. Brace yourself for a profound revelation: the diffused artwork of isometrics, whilst blended with aware practices including meditation, has the functionality not only to relieve stress however additionally to elevate cognizance and mental nicely-being. Can the energy to lessen stress and beautify attention actually be located within the global of isometric sporting activities? Let's delve into the intricacies of this captivating connection and find the transformative effect it is able to need on your traditional nicely-being.

Discovering Harmony

Within the scope of isometric wearing sports for women, the symbiotic dating among the mind and frame performs a pivotal function in accomplishing holistic nicely-being. In this segment, we will delve into the profound impact of incorporating meditation into isometric sports sports.

Understanding the Harmony amongst Mind and Body

The fusion of meditation and isometric physical video games creates a effective synergy that transcends the bodily realm. Isometric sports comprise contracting muscle tissues with out changing their period, promoting each energy and staying power. Simultaneously, meditation cultivates a serene intellectual country, fostering emotional stability and mindfulness.

Unveiling the Mental Benefits

1. Stress Reduction: Isometric bodily sports, at the equal time as determined by meditation, act as a effective stress-treatment duo. Stress

regularly manifests physical, inflicting muscle tension and soreness. Engaging in isometrics on the same time as preserving a meditative mind-set alleviates strain with the resource of selling muscle rest and highbrow tranquility.

2. Enhanced Focus: Meditation enhances awareness, a potential at once relevant to isometric carrying sports. The mindful method finally of isometrics lets in you focus at an appropriate muscle agencies being engaged, refining your thoughts-muscle connection. This heightened cognizance contributes to better form, advanced overall performance, and advanced consequences.

The How-To of Meditative Isometrics

1. Setting the Scene: Find a quiet place wherein you could carry out your isometric bodily sports activities without distractions. Begin with some deep breaths to middle your self and transition into a meditative nation.

2. Mindful Muscle Engagement: As you keep with isometric carrying sports, awareness on

the targeted muscle institution. Picture the muscle jogging, contracting, and liberating. This intellectual imagery not handiest deepens your reference to your body but additionally intensifies the effectiveness of the sports activities sports.

3. Breath Awareness: Sync your breath along side your isometric moves. Inhale at some point of the muscle contraction segment and exhale throughout the relaxation section. This rhythmic respiration now not most effective enhances oxygen flow to the muscles however furthermore promotes a calming impact on your nerve-racking tool.

The Scientific Backing

Research has confirmed that combining isometric sports with meditation induces high-quality changes within the thoughts. The dual effect at the thoughts and frame enables lessen cortisol ranges, the hormone associated with strain. Additionally, the release of endorphins, brought on by using the use of way of every sports activities, contributes to an regular experience of properly-being.

Incorporating Meditation into Your Routine

To embody the fusion of meditation and isometric physical sports activities, bear in mind dedicating a couple of minutes to mindfulness in advance than or after your exercise training. Experiment with honestly one in every of a type meditation strategies, along with guided imagery or mindfulness meditation, to find out what resonates nice with you.

By intertwining the ones practices, you now not handiest sculpt a stronger body however additionally nurture a resilient and serene mind. As you embark on this transformative journey, maintain in thoughts that the course to well being includes the harmonious balance of both body and mind.

Unraveling the Benefits: Stress Reduction and Improved Focus

In the pursuit of widespread well-being thru isometric bodily games for ladies, Chapter nine.2 delves deeper into the profound impact the ones carrying sports have on strain good buy and consciousness improvement. The interconnectedness among physical interest and highbrow readability bureaucracy a cornerstone for engaging in a balanced and quality way of life.

The Stress-Reduction Power of Isometric Exercises

1. Muscle Relaxation: Isometric wearing activities inherently contain contracting muscle mass without joint movement, leading to muscle relaxation. This physical release of hysteria extends beyond the muscle groups, influencing the concerned tool to unwind. As a stop cease end result, the exercise of isometrics will become a restoration treatment for the amassed stress of each day lifestyles.

2. Cortisol Regulation: Isometric carrying activities play a critical characteristic in

regulating cortisol, the body's number one stress hormone. Engaging in the ones sporting events activates the discharge of endorphins, which counteract the effects of cortisol. This hormonal equilibrium contributes to a more serene intellectual kingdom, fostering resilience towards stressors.

Improved Focus via Isometric Exercises

1. Mind-Muscle Connection: Isometric bodily sports call for a heightened recognition of the muscle companies being engaged. This intentional reputation on precise muscle businesses complements the mind-muscle connection, sharpening your awareness at some stage in sporting events. The planned intellectual engagement in every exercise cultivates a revel in of mindfulness, redirecting your interest away from out of doors stressors.

2. Neuroplasticity Enhancement: Regular isometric carrying sports stimulate neuroplasticity – the brain's capability to comply and reorganize. This adaptability

extends to cognitive functions, which includes hobby and consciousness. As you commonly engage in isometrics, your brain office work new neural connections that contribute to advanced hobby and cognitive flexibility.

Implementing Stress Reduction and Improved Focus in Your Routine

1. Structured Workouts: Incorporate isometric wearing occasions strategically within your exercise everyday. Begin with a warm-as plenty as put together your muscles, then seamlessly transition into isometrics. As you development, pay aware attention to the feeling in each muscle employer, permitting the sporting activities to end up a aware exercise.

www.ingramcontent.com/pod-product-compliance
Lightning Source LLC
La Vergne TN
LVHW021053071025
822752LV00029B/111